Positive Pregnancy Fitness

A Guide to a More Comfortable Pregnancy and
Easier Birth Through Exercise and Relaxation

Sylvia Klein Olkin, M.S.

Technical Advisor Carl Mailhot

Drawings by Antonia

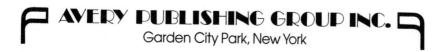
AVERY PUBLISHING GROUP INC.
Garden City Park, New York

Cover Design by Rudy Shur and Martin Hochberg
Cover Art by Tim Peterson
Drawings by Antonia
In-House Editor Jacqueline Balla

With love to my sons, Mathew and Michael,
and to all future babies of the world.
May they have the power and courage
to make the world a more
peaceful and productive place.

Olkin, Sylvia Klein.
    Positive pregnancy fitness.

    Bibliography: p.
    Includes indexes.
    1. Pregnancy. 2. Exercise for women.
3. Physical fitness for women. I. Title.
[DNLM: 1. Exertion—in pregnancy—popular
works. 2. Physical Fitness—popular works.
3. Pregnancy—popular works. 4. Relaxation
Technics—in pregnancy—popular works.
WQ   150   049p]
RG558.7.O427   1987   618.2 ′4   87-18844
ISBN 0-89529-373-0 (soft)

Printed in the United States of America

10 9 8 7 6 5 4 3

Contents

Acknowledgements

The creation, development, and completion of this book would not have been possible without the generous efforts of a special group of people. My sincere thanks to:

My husband, Bob, and our sons, Mathew and Michael, for their encouragement and faith when the "going got tough" right after my stroke. I will never forget their constant concern and caring.

My parents, Nora and Meyer Klein, for their caring and support. They had faith in me and believed that I could learn to read and write all over again, even though I didn't think that this was possible at the time. Naturally, they were right!

My sister, Helaine Ronen, who was always there when I needed her the most.

My whole family, for their concern, unrelenting telephone calls, and visits of support. They knew that I would somehow have the power and strength to heal my body.

My yoga teachers, Bob and Thelma Peck, for providing the "spark" that led to the writing of this book, and for being the kind of people who continually share their time, love, and enthusiasm for life.

The Monday and Tuesday night meditation classes, for giving me encouragement and energy.

Antonia, whose illustrations have helped this book to come alive with vitality, gracefulness, and joy. The door is always open.

Sandra Lucas, for her original chakra and herbal drawings.

Jan Allard, Teresa Bonillo, and Tonia Shaevitz, who patiently read and corrected the manuscript, especially during the time when I couldn't write or spell.

Jacquie Burzychi, R.N., Positive Parenting Fitness Master Teacher, and Sean Burzychi, her unborn child, who patiently posed for the hundreds of photos on which the illustrations in this book are based. Many thanks also to Keith Burzychi for posing for the massage photos.

Naomi and David Howe, for being the kind of friends I could always count on. Their continuous support and editorial comments during the preparation of this book were invaluable.

Nancy and Paul Cohen, for being steadfast friends and caring, loving, and supportive people.

May Ellen O'Hara, Ph.D, Positive Pregnancy Fitness Master Teacher, who contributed the original ideas for the chapter, *Prenatal Psychology and "Inner Bonding."* Mary Ellen has always been there when I needed her the most with helpful ideas, suggestions, and genuine caring.

Mary Grady, Positive Pregnancy Fitness Master Teacher, who developed the PPF Wet Program described in this book. Special thanks to Mary for being a super teacher whose enthusiasm for the PPF approach is highly contagious.

Sharon Lopez, yoga teacher and PPF Master Teacher, who has contributed so much to the development of PPF.

Grace Burkhardt, RN, PPF instructor, who contributed her knowledge of shiatsu pressure points for labor to the chapter on massage and has been extremely helpful and knowledgeable in a variety of areas.

Adair Luciano, PPF instructor, who contributed the original idea of using a tangible leaf for the chapter on fear.

Carl Mailhot, B.S., R.P.T., whose technical expertise and suggestions have added so much to this book.

Carroll Mailhot, PPF Certified Teacher, for picking me up when I was down.

Dr. Frank Carter, for his practical and helpful medical advice and for his support and encouragement when I needed it the most.

Beth Carter, for her editorial assistance and ideas.

Frederick Leboyer, for his enlightening correspondence on "inner bonding."

Linda Green, R.N., D.P.A., for her helpful research on the physiology of pregnancy and birth.

Terri Mooney, RN, International Board Certified Lactation Consultant (IBCLC), for her useful suggestions regarding nursing.

Nan Ullrike Koehler, M.S., botanist, for her expert advice on herbs.

Charis Tondreau and David Engler, Registered Therapeutic Massage Therapists, for their expert advice and suggestions on massage.

Gerry Impallomeni and Rosemary Mazor, PPF and certified aerobic fitness instructors, who contributed to the weight training chapter.

Rudy Shur, Managing Editor at Avery, who waited a very, very long time for the completion of this book, but was super supportive and understanding.

Jacqueline Balla, my editor at Avery, for doing such a good job in editing this book.

The hundreds of Positive Pregnancy Fitness teachers across the country who said prayers for me, sent along healing energy, or wrote encouraging letters at a time when I thought I would never complete this book.

All the future mothers, fathers, and babies of the world. I wish you peace, joy, and love.

Foreword

I have practiced obstetrics and gynecology for over twenty-five years, and have noticed that women would like to be more informed and active participants in their pregnancies. Sylvia Klein Olkin's book, *Positive Pregnancy Fitness*, is a fascinating and practical approach to the preparation for pregnancy, labor, and delivery.

Sylvia Klein Olkin has been interested in yoga for many years and has taught at a variety of places, from Connecticut College to the local YMCA. She has combined her own personal experience with her knowledge of yoga to develop special classes for the management of prepared childbirth. I have known Sylvia for a number of years, and it has been a pleasure to see the expertise and feeling she brings to the woman who is trying to prepare herself for pregnancy, labor, and delivery. Sylvia has carefully researched her information and has sought expert advice on the subjects that are included in her book. I am also very excited by the fact that she has been sponsoring PPF teacher-training workshops throughout the country, so that interested childbirth educators will be exposed to a holistic approach to pregnancy.

Positive Pregnancy Fitness is a useful book I would recommend to all my patients to help them to have a happy and successful childbearing experience.

Frank J. Carter, M.D.
President of the Staff
Senior, Department of OB/GYN
Wm. W. Backus Hospital
Norwich, Connecticut
Assistant Clinical Professor
School of Nursing, Yale University

Preface

Life is full of ironic twists. I attended my first yoga class to get rid of a backache I had endured all during my second pregnancy and for a year following the birth of my son, Mike. Little did I know I would someday be teaching pregnant women how to leave their pain behind and feel good during pregnancy, in a yoga program designed especially for the mother-to-be.

As I began the research that would one day evolve into the PPF (Positive Pregnancy Fitness) program, I read many books and talked with numerous doctors, nurses, midwives, physical therapists, psychologists, professors of obstetrical nursing, and many, many pregnant women. I began to understand which parts of the pregnant body needed to be specially prepared for birth, and the need for relaxation skills for a positive birth experience. Even more importantly, I began to explore the mental space of pregnancy.

I will never forget teaching my first prenatal class. After so much researching, thinking, wondering, and talking, here I was facing fifteen real live pregnant women! As I was about to begin, small index cards filled with exercise directions in my hands, I looked around at the faces of my students. They were not quite sure what to expect and, to a certain extent, neither was I. I happened to look around the room for a second time and this time I could have sworn that I saw another set of eyes—wide-open, tiny eyes—looking back at me! It was at this moment that the duality of pregnancy became very real to me. I realized I would be working with a double audience and everything that I included in my program would have to be beneficial for each set of partners. I was engulfed with a feeling of sheer panic. Was I really prepared? Would all fifteen women and their babies feel better after the class had ended? Were the exercises we would practice that day as safe and useful as I thought them to be? With these questions and others racing through my frenzied mind, I quickly decided to immediately teach the women how to breathe abdominally so their teacher could calm down and center! The deep breathing turned panic into a calmness and frenzy into faith, and the PPF program was launched.

It is a continually rewarding experience to spend time and share space with pregnant women. There is a special feeling—a special energy—a special love in these groups. In fact, the most useful information in this book was discovered or created in my PPF classes. The exercises, breathing techniques, and relaxation/visualizations have been "people-tested" and thereby proven safe and effective, and have produced positive and lasting results.

At the request of a very persistent childbirth educator from Maine, I began holding teacher training workshops in my home. To date, I have traveled across the United States and Canada teaching two-day PPF Teacher-Training Workshops in hotels and hospitals. I have worked with over 600 enthusiastic, caring, and dedicated childbirth educators, nurses, midwives, physical therapists, and yoga teachers, teaching them about prenatal fitness. Amazing as it may seem, I learn something new at every workshop.

Suddenly, in the spring of 1985, my health completely deteriorated. I contracted Myasthenia Gravis, a severe neurological disease, and had a series of strokes. The Myasthenia left me with extremely weak muscles that didn't always function properly. Because of the strokes I couldn't speak, read, or write.

Should I give up my dreams of sharing valuable PPF exercises and information just because I had suffered some severe setbacks? Maybe the sensible approach would have been to give up the PPF Teacher Training Workshops, and call up my publisher and ask for an indefinite extension of this manuscript.

But I sensed that if I gave up my dreams and goals, no matter how difficult they had become to achieve, I would lose my zest for living. I tried to formulate a sensible plan to keep the PPF Teacher Training Workshops going.

Luckily I have been surrounded and encouraged by incredibly supportive people— Mary Ellen O'Hara, Mary Grady, Sharon Lopez, and Jacquie Burzycki. They took over my PPF workshops so I could concentrate on getting well.

I took speech therapy to improve my pronunciation and physical therapy to relearn how to use my right hand. When your brain cells are destroyed as a result of a stroke, you still have the capacity to relearn various things. You simply have to take the time and effort to reprogram your brain.

My family and teachers were so supportive and understanding, I really couldn't feel sorry for myself. It seemed an enormous undertaking just to regain the little things in life that we all take for granted. I was really frustrated. So what did I do?

I followed the PPF program—I meditated every day, did whatever yoga I could (in the beginning it was very little indeed) and breathed deeply whenever I felt utter frustration at not being able to express myself. Most importantly, I awoke every day with the positive attitude that, in time, I would regain all my faculties. There are some days, I have to admit, when the Myasthenia acts up and I am so weak that I feel like giving up. But I immediately go back to my PPF disciplines: meditation, nutritious food, and exercise blended with a large dose of faith. I have gotten progressively better, and my faith in the PPF program has sustained me.

Throughout your pregnancy you, too, will be facing different challenges in your life. The PPF program will help expand your understanding of pregnancy. There is still so much to discover and explore about the pregnancy and birth process. Because most of the childbirth education programs of the past have focused only on the last 6-8 weeks of pregnancy, we are exploring a vast new span of time and experience.

I have tried to make this book as personal as possible in order to duplicate the personal attention given to PPF students. I hope that you will be able to find a PPF teacher in your community. If not, I invite you to become my student via this book. I know that the fitness program contained in this book can help you to harmonize your inner and outer worlds, thereby enabling you to more fully enjoy and experience pregnancy and motherhood. I hope that the seasons of your life—summer, fall, winter, and spring—will be times of inner and outer growth, strength, and discovery.

Joy,
Sylvia

Introduction

Pregnancy is a blessed state of consciousness. It is unique and even scary sometimes. We are only now beginning to realize the depths and possibilities of this beautiful time in life. Therefore, this book is only a beginning exploration of a very complex, multifaceted time in a woman's life.

Pregnancy is like walking into the unknown. It is a time of growth—physical, mental, and spiritual. It is a time full of rich meaning. It is a fruitful time. It is a significant time. It is a mentally-fertile time, full of ideas and daydreams.

Pregnancy is a time of transition. It is a time of lost self-images. It is a time of doubt. It is a time of future commitment. It is a time of physical aches and abuses. It is a time of laughter and tears. It is a time of union. It is the only time in your life when your consciousness and the consciousness of your unborn child are housed in one body.

Pregnancy is a time of physical miracles. It is a time of the daily physical change necessary to accommodate both you and your baby. It is a time of increased blood volume necessary to feed and oxygenate your baby while your own body still thrives. It is a time of increased demand on all your bodily systems. It is a time to be in tune with the natural knowledge and rhythms within your body.

Pregnancy is an opening, both physically and mentally. Your rib cage opens to increase oxygen intake; your pelvic bones spread open to enable the baby to pass through in the process of birth. Your mind is also open to new thoughts, new ideas, new inner awarenesses.

Pregnancy is a contradiction. It is a time of daydreams, fantasies, and expectations. But it is also a time of inward searching, inward dwelling, and inward exploration.

Pregnancy is your time. Nature has provided you with the time to help you ease from one being into two. It is your own personal experience. Some segments of your experience will be described in the many books and articles on the topic. But the essence of the experience, on its various levels of your being and consciousness, is your own personal path. Womanhood has graced you with a transition stage that enables you to grow into parenthood. Open your eyes and become aware that we have nine months in which to slowly grow, evolve, nourish, sustain, and ultimately give birth to a new life.

Pregnancy is the perfect time to pursue a self-development program that works with your natural inclinations. Working with and understanding your own processes and functions will add greater depth to your pregnancy experience. It can truly become a smooth period of transition from which you will discover your own untapped inner knowledge, inner strength, and inner wisdom.

Part I
Positive Pregnancy Fitness

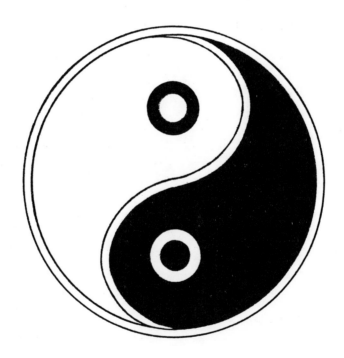

Yin-Yang, Chinese symbol of duality in Nature:
"Perfect Action and Strength, Perfect Stillness and Concentration."

CHAPTER ONE
Positive Pregnancy Fitness

Life can be an intriguing teacher, especially when you are pregnant. Your old world will very often take on new meaning because of the life that is growing and being nurtured inside you. There is a natural tendency to search for new insights, new data, and new facts that will shape the kind of pregnancy you have. *Positive Pregnancy Fitness* takes into account the total person that you are. It is holistic in the sense that it works with the way you feel, your reaction to stress, your daily emotions, prenatal bonding with your baby, and much more. It contains safe exercises that will enhance your comfort level throughout your pregnancy.

Pregnancy fitness means a wholeness in the way you view yourself, your pregnancy, and your baby. It means developing yourself in special ways so that you will take time for yourself and your needs. For if you can center yourself and understand why you are going through certain changes, you are sure to grow in essential ways along your journey to motherhood.

The PPF program grew out of the "pregnancy frame of mind" I discovered as I explored the world of pregnancy from my students' viewpoints. As we freely exchanged information, I began to learn about my students' dreams, ideas, questions, observations, and various other facets of the pregnancy experience. I spent numerous hours exploring this "pregnancy space" while gathering information for the PPF program.

As the PPF program evolved, I was to find out that pregnancy affects every part of your life. Although I started out teaching a simple one-hour exercise class for pregnant women ten years ago, today the program consists of exercise, stress management, relaxation/visualization and other information that is taught in over thirty states.

PPF: AN OVERVIEW

In order to explore the entire pregnancy experience, I've included visualization exercises that you should try on your own to help you to become more in touch with your baby. There is a very large chapter devoted to safe prenatal exercises that will insure comfort and reduce stress during all facets of your pregnancy. These physical exercises will invigorate you after a busy day. Building a healthy baby also requires a healthy diet, so a chapter has been devoted to nutrition. Two chapters have been devoted to exploring the moods and fears of pregnancy. There is just so much to explore and understand about pregnancy—it is almost as big as life itself!

My training as a yoga teacher has influenced my approach to pregnancy and new life. I realized ten years ago that a combination of yoga and knowledge of the pregnancy experience would serve a very important function. If my students could understand why they felt a certain way and be able to learn how to make themselves feel better, then a positive and useful contribution could be made to the whole pregnancy experience. It is this "marriage" of the discipline of yoga and the entire pregnancy experience that is the goal of this book. If you faithfully practice the PPF program once every day or even every other day, a better pregnancy is almost guaranteed.

HOW OUR BRAINS FUNCTION

Yoga training involves finding a balance between our rational selves and our intuitive selves. Our tendency is to overwork the rational, outer-directed, programmed part of the brain, while simply ignoring the inner-directed, intuitive, creative side. Learning to build pathways between the two halves of our brains can only increase our potential and overall enjoyment of life.

Figure 1.1 is a representation of the *Split Brain Theory* that explains the different functions served by the left and right hemispheres of your brain. In studying Figure 1.1, you will notice that the left side is thought to control our rational and outer-directed selves. This side deals with such processes as linear thinking, verbal and routine memory, logical thought, mechanical and analytical thinking, and action that goes with our thoughts. The right side is thought to control our irrational and inner-directed selves. This side of the brain deals with intuition, our artistic and creative selves, spatial relations, meditative spaces, visual images, and aesthetics. Getting these two very different parts of ourselves to work together in harmony is what the PPF program is all about.

Since we are a society that is based largely on scientific research, is it any wonder that we tend to ignore the right side of the brain? We are constantly doing things, studying things, analyzing things, enjoying things. In addition, we like to believe that everything in our lives is rational and logical. So we tend to ignore any sinking feeling that threatens danger.

Figure 1.1   The Split Brain*

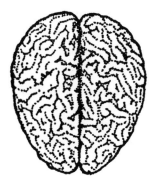

Left Brain **	Right Brain
(Right Side of Body)	(Left Side of Body)
Rational	Irrational
Outer-directed	Inner-directed
Speech/Verbal	Spatial/Musical
Programmed	Holistic
Logical/Mathematical	Artistic/Symbolic
Linear/Detailed	Simultaneous
Controlled	Emotional
Intellectual	Intuitive/Creative
Dominant	Spiritual/Oneness
Active	Receptive
Analytic	Visual
Reading/Writing/Naming	Acceptance
Sequential ordering	Infinite
	Feeling
Complex Order	
Complex Motor Sequences	Perceptions of Abstract Patterns
	Recognition of Abstract Figures

In my research I've noticed an altered state of consciousness—superconsciousness, so to speak—when a woman desperately wants to tune in to the ignored right hemisphere of the brain. The PPF program encourages you to tune into your body and your baby. It maximizes your enjoyment of pregnancy with stretching and breathing exercises that keep you in touch with your baby through "inner bonding" techniques. In addition, PPF offers you natural tips for eliminating the annoyances and discomforts of pregnancy. Most importantly, it encourages you to have a positive outlook on life throughout your pregnancy.

I suggest that once you learn the exercises in this book, you close your eyes and tune it on to what you are experiencing inside. Available to you, there are three audio tapes that accompany the program: *Positive Pregnancy Fitness, Breathing for Birth,* and *Relax and Enjoy Your Baby Within* (see the Appendix).

---

*This representation of the *split brain theory* is based on findings printed in *American Meditation and Beginning Yoga* by Robert L. Peck (1976) and the *Bulletin of the Theosopy Science Group,* India, December, 1976.

**Note that in a few people the functions are reversed.

YOGA AND PREGNANCY

You may gain a better understanding of the yoga philosophy on which PPF is based by using your imagination. For example, imagine that you are looking at a still photograph of a lovely tropical scene. In your mind's eye, envision the palm trees, the white sandy beach, the colorful flowers, vines, and trees. Further embellish this mental picture with a deep blue cloudless sky, the blue-green waters of a calm lagoon bathed in golden sunshine. See the variety of people on the beach: two small children digging in the sand, a young man reading, an older couple playing cards, two teenagers lazily swimming in the calm water. A small sailboat is on the horizon and its inhabitants are waving to the young man on the beach. Try to make this scene as real as you can.

Now let's make this scene even more real and exciting by turning it into a moving picture. Mentally see the palm trees blowing and bending lazily in the breeze as the people begin to move about doing their own activities. See the children constructing a large sand city. They have already built the smaller buildings and are now working on the main castle with a high elaborate moat. One child is going to fill his bucket with water for the moat around the castle. Hear the sounds of the warm calm water lapping lazily onto the beach as the birds' chirping blends with the sounds of undistinguishable conversations on the beach. Several new people are coming onto the beach: mentally see who they are and what they are doing. Try to make yourself a part of this moving picture by imagining how you would feel if you were in this very beautiful scene. Imagine how the scene would smell, sound, and feel to you.

You may be wondering by now what the connection is between these scenes and the study of yoga. The connection is really quite simple. Life without yoga can be compared to a still photograph of a place. You can see all the parts of the scene, but there is no action. You may be content with this still view of life, but there really is more for you to explore and experience. The discipline of yoga can enable you to fully experience and enjoy the various levels of your life. By learning more about how you function—your brain and your body—you will learn to heighten your senses, thereby deepening your daily experiences. You will, in essence, become more alive. It may seem illogical to you for a "discipline" to give you enjoyment and pleasure. People usually think of "discipline" as punishment or something to be avoided at all costs. We discipline our children when they exhibit unacceptable behavior. From a yogic point of view, "discipline" is the application of yogic rules and exercises to all aspects of life. By merely integrating yogic practices into your daily routine, you will begin to notice things about yourself that you were not aware of before. When you begin to notice things about yourself, you begin to notice new things about people and the outside world as well. With the excitement, anxiety, and expectancy of a new baby growing inside you, the benefits to be derived from practicing yoga are varied and large.

Use your imagination once again and come with me to one of my Positive Pregnancy Fitness classes. It is the first class of an eight-week series, and the new students are walking down the brightly-lit corridor carrying their blankets, pillows, and purses, looking for the meeting room. Some of the women are walking with the pregnancy waddle of the later months; others are just beginning to show. Once my new students have found the room and are settled on their mats, lively conversation inevitably begins. If you listen closely, you can hear someone asking, "When are you due?" or "How much weight have you gained so far?" or "You have a backache, too?"

There is a special feeling in this room. A feeling of anticipation, of expectancy, of heightened energy. Each woman is here to prepare herself for a very important event: the birth of her baby, and of a new consciousness. She wants to be in good physical, mental, and emotional shape in order to enhance her birthing experience. I am sure you want these same things, too.

When I begin the class with each woman introducing herself and announcing her due date, it is always fun to see which women will be having their babies at the same time of year. Next comes the barrage of questions; there are always so many on the first evening of class. "What kind of exercises should I *not* be doing?" "Can I continue to jog?" "What is a well-balanced diet anyhow?" "What does yoga have to do with having a baby?" Maybe you have one to ask. This is only a brief sampling of the many questions asked and answered during this class session. These women want simple answers and remedies to the everyday complaints and experiences of pregnancy. And they want the answers *fast,* for their time is limited and they have a lot to learn before their babies arrive.

I explain that an ancient system of self-discipline has the answers for which they have been searching. At this point someone usually asks, "What is yoga?" You may be curious about this question as well. The best way to explain yoga is to say that it is a highly scientific system for self-improvement and self-knowledge. The word "yoga" comes from an ancient Indian language called Sanskrit. It is derived from the verbal root "yuk," which literally means to "yoke, join together, or unite." The yogic system, if practiced correctly, can allow the student to experience the union of the mind and the body and, eventually, union with the Universal Spirit. The term "hatha," which describes the physical aspect of yoga, literally means sun (ha) and moon (tha). This is symbolic of the warm and cool aspects of each individual that can be integrated by the practice of physical yoga. This integration can lead to an even flow of energy through the body's channels, as well as increased good health. Mental and physical harmony are the goals achieved by consistent practice. By combining the physical system with some forms of controlled breathing, relaxation and/or meditation, you can contribute to your own development and perfection—both physically and spiritually.

After this rather deep philosophical explanation of hatha yoga and how it works, a student often asks, "But what does all this stuff have to do with having a baby?" That is a very valid question, and if you think about the foregoing information for a moment, you may begin to have a glimmer of what yoga is all about. Remember that the word yoga means union. When you are pregnant, it is the only time in your life that you are experiencing a daily physical union with another being. Your body and that of the baby are continually interconnected. The baby is dependent on you throughout its development. Thus you are actually experiencing a form of union or yoga while you are pregnant. It is very different from what is generally described in the ancient yogic writings, but it *is* one level of yoga nonetheless. Since you are in such a close relationship with your future child, if you take the time to learn control of your body and your mind while you are pregnant, it will be exceedingly beneficial for the baby growing within. Your baby is extremely sensitive to your ups and downs.

Finally, it is time to stretch into our first yoga asana, or exercise. Here is another Sanskrit word that describes the special kind of movements which are the cornerstone of a physical yoga program. *Asana* is a position which is easy and comfortable, as well as firm. This means going into a stretch, keeping your mind on the feelings it is giving you, and holding it for as long as is comfortable. You may want to imagine that you are a member of this imaginary class right now and try your first PPF exercise with us. Read these directions over twice before trying this simple arm stretch. It is very important for inner centering that you keep your eyes closed and feel your body move.

Simple Arm Stretch

1. Lift your arms up slowly above your head.
2. Feel your arm muscles tightening as you move.
3. Clasp your hands together, turn the palms toward the ceiling, and stretch.
4. Breathe normally, as you mentally feel your arms stretching and your rib cage moving up.
5. Hold for as long as is comfortable and then slowly float the arms back down to your sides.

If you observe yourself carefully, you will find that your body will automatically take a breath once your arms return to your sides. It is now time to learn to take a deep PPF abdominal breath. Here again you must concentrate mentally on every bodily movement as we all deep breathe together.

PPF Abdominal Breath

1. Place your hands on the baby area.
2. Relax the tummy.
3. Inhale through the nose and move the tummy (baby) forward.
4. Immediately exhale through the nose and move the tummy (baby) back.
5. Repeat this breath again.

This breath will both balance out the stretch and wash carbon dioxide from your muscles so you do not ache later.

This deep breath is followed by many new and interesting stretches as the prenatal physical program unfolds. Finally, time has slipped away and the end of class is nearing. After all the new bends and stretches of the PPF program, most students are only too glad to get into a comfortable position and relax their minds and bodies completely for several minutes. Once this relaxation is complete and the students are beginning to move again, any earlier restlessness is gone and has been replaced by an inner calm. Many new yoga students have commented that they really do not fully understand life with a yogic slant, but they do know it feels terrific.

You can join this group of students by participating in my prenatal classes via this book. If you take some private time each day to come into my classroom, your senses will be heightened, your worries eased, and your total enjoyment of life increased. Yoga will not eliminate trouble from your life, but it will help you to see things from a new perspective so that you can live life to its fullest at this very exciting time. The joy in life is there for the taking. It is doubled when you are pregnant! There is joy in the little things which you may have missed before. Taking a deep breath and feeling the extra vitality in your body feels wonderful. Maybe your baby will kick and say "thank-you" for the extra boost of energy he received. From a yogic point of view, life is to be enjoyed and experienced to the fullest. There is so much to see, taste, feel, hear, and know. Life is full of movement, vitality, and change, just as in a moving picture. Don't miss all the action by not paying attention to it while you think or worry about what could happen or what happened ten years ago. Once you learn to quiet your mind and tune into your body and baby, you can truly begin to experience and enjoy the beautiful world in which we live.

CHAPTER TWO
Stress Management During Pregnancy

"Why do I feel so unsettled and upset all the time?" asked a first-time mother at the end of one of my early PPF classes. "Why didn't someone tell me that all the changes during pregnancy were not only physical? I am just not thinking and reacting the way I used to before my pregnancy. Is there something wrong with me?" I spent the next hour discovering that my student was feeling stress and couldn't handle it very well.

I was given a lot of insight into the ongoing myriad of changes that were affecting every level of her body and mind. Some of the changes had been welcomed, such as the change in her body shape to accommodate the growing baby, and feeling her baby kick for the first time. But many of the changes puzzled her because by the time she had gotten used to them, they either disappeared or changed. The most confusing of all were her mental reactions to everyday occurrences. She found herself reacting with new intensity—both positive and negative—to daily happenings, to movies she saw, to people she met. It was as if she were seeing life in a new way, and this really upset her. As her state of consciousness became clearer, I realized that the relationship between stress and pregnancy had to be further studied and explored. My basic goal was to find methods that would help pregnant women to calm down and regain control when they found themselves under intense stress. Before exploring the techniques that we discovered, however, it might be helpful for you to acquire a better understanding of stress and how it affects you.

WHAT IS STRESS?

Many of today's health practitioners and medical researchers have designated stress as the "Disease of the 80's"—one of the most debilitating medical and social problems in the country today. It is quite different from other diseases because it has no biological basis such as a germ or a virus. Rather, it is a direct result of how our minds and bodies function and interact together. The way in which you regulate your mental and physical functioning determines your level of stress. It is your conscious or unconscious choices in daily living that ultimately dictate your stress level.

The factors that lead to a stressed or unbalanced mind and body are many. Emotional or mental stress is a result of your interaction with your daily environment and includes the people you relate with, as well as your physical surroundings. Several examples of this type of stress would include daily mishaps, fears that are unrealized, worries about the future, and concerns about what the neighbors would think of something you have done or might do.

Digestive stress results from poor or erratic eating habits, which tax the body's ability to digest and absorb the elements necessary for good health. Environmental stress is created by environments which are innundated with smog, noise, or air pollution.

It is upsetting to realize that people suffer headaches, stomach aches, and physical aches and pains as a result of their choice of lifestyles. In order to cope with these situations, many nonpregnant people often treat or mask stress by smoking, drinking, taking aspirin or sleeping pills, or even taking a vacation. But any kind of escape is only temporary, and inevitably you have to face the hassles and upsets of daily life.

Once you realize that you cannot change many of the stressors of daily life, it becomes clear that it is your own physical and mental reactions to these situations that *can and should be changed.* Learning how to change your own reactions to stress—both physical and mental—takes a lot of hard work and basic stress management guidelines. Making this decision when you are pregnant is an especially wise choice, since many of the outlets people choose to escape from stress, such as smoking and drinking, are detrimental to your baby's mental and physical development.

THE STRESS OF PREGNANCY

We know from studies on stress conducted in 1976 by T.H. Holmes and R.H. Rahe that life events can be ranked according to social impact. These studies found pregnancy to be the 12th most stressful life event, following other traumatic events such as the death of a spouse (#1), divorce (#2), the loss of a job (#8) and others. Many newly-pregnant women are not aware that the forthcoming nine months may indeed be one of the most stressful periods of their lives. Many factors—including changes in personal perception, changes in body image, anxiety about future responsibilities, changes in sexual response, and others—contribute to stress during the transition period of pregnancy.

Although your own individual reactions to pregnancy will be unique, you may find that you have a lot of feelings in common with other pregnant women. Research has shown that women often go through many specific responses during the three trimesters (or 3-month segments) of pregnancy. You'll probably sigh with relief when you learn that your own responses *have* been experienced by other women in your situation.

The First Trimester

During the first trimester of pregnancy, emotional responses often include:

- a sense of estrangement or detachment
- mood swings ranging from joy to sadness
- decreased sexual interest
- ambivalence about the pregnancy
- beginning change in body image

Although there may be few outward changes to indicate the existence of pregnancy, many women experience morning sickness, tiredness, tenderness of the breasts, and other physical discomforts which may increase levels of stress. Some of these discomforts can be minimized or even completely eliminated with the natural techniques recommended in Chapter 4. Others will disappear with the continuation of the pregnancy.

The Second Trimester

Your baby will become real to you in the second trimester as you begin to feel movement and life within. When your baby kicks or moves for the first time, this tangible experience will intensify the reality of your condition. These three months are typically characterized as the "quiet months" and many women may experience:

- a sense of enhanced well-being
- heightened body awareness
- heightened sexual awareness
- awareness that you cannot control your body's changes
- introversion over future mothering role
- heightened anxieties and/or phobias

It is at this time in your pregnancy that you may want to share your thoughts and feelings with other women. Check to see if there are any PPF classes offered in your community. You will find the support and understanding of the other women in your class to be invaluable.

The Third Trimester

During these three months your body will continue to enlarge and change as you continue to adapt. Some of the experiences associated with the third trimester are:

- physical discomfort
- changes in sexuality

- •mental expectation about life with a new baby
- •increased anxiety over the unknown future
- •decreased self-esteem if the woman stops working
- •fear of losing control
- •a distorted body image
- •conflicts caused by shifts from dependence to independence

By the end of the third trimester, you may feel that "enough is enough" and long for the end of pregnancy and the start of your new mothering role.

LABOR, DELIVERY, AND PARENTHOOD

All of the changes, anxieties, pleasures, and expectations are crowned with the actual birth of your child. Birth is an emotional and physical experience of unparalleled intensity. In fact, it can be and often is a turning point in your life. The stresses of birth are both mental and physical. Your body works with your baby, pushing and finally easing your child out to meet you. The intensity of the pain and mental and physical effort involved can and often does tap all of your resources.

Once you are face to face with your baby, you will find new stressors to keep your life quite busy. You will have to adjust to the strains and pressures of motherhood as you accept the various tasks involved. You will have to care for an infant on very little sleep and with a body that is still healing. Attention to your child's development and needs will have to be balanced with your own personal sense of autonomy. More importantly, you will have to make satisfactory adjustments to the realities of life. Raising a child takes a lot of hard work.

Some of this information may be causing your stress right now as you read about it. You may be wondering how you will be able to cope with it all. But whatever you do, don't close the book and give up at this point, because help is on the way! You might even end up having fun and enjoying the whole experience!

SELF-MANAGEMENT FOR STRESS REDUCTION

Since you have the ability—on many different levels—to react to the experience of pregnancy, birth, and parenting in a variety of ways, you also have the capacity to teach yourself how to better deal with your own powerful reactions. There are some specific techniques that will enable you to control your emotions and thoughts, but remember that the PPF program as a whole is designed to keep you and the child within you healthy and strong.

Because you may be feeling more stress since your pregnancy began, this is a good time to explore a holistic or multi-faceted approach for handling the situation. Let's outline the different aspects of your life that need to be analyzed and changed to help you better cope with stress in your life.

To reduce the stress in your life, you need to be aware of useful stress management techniques including:

•regular daily exercise
•healthful nutrition
•letting-go techniques, such as controlled breathing and meditation
•self-awareness and faith in yourself
•personal planning

Although breathing techniques are powerful tools for teaching you to control your mind and body, there are other techniques that can help, too. As more and more people are becoming aware of the connection between daily exercise and good health, they are also discovering that exercise has a very beneficial effect on reducing stress levels. Chapter 7 contains a varied program of exercises that can be used every day of your pregnancy. In addition, you should be walking between one and two miles a day. Incorporating a weekly swimming program into your schedule will also add an aerobic factor to your exercise routines.

Your Diet

Your daily diet during the nine months of pregnancy will determine how you feel and the health of your baby. If you suffer from morning sickness or nausea early in your pregnancy, you may not want to even think about food. But as soon as the first trimester is over, the nausea usually disappears and you can begin to make decisions regarding your stress level and health. Chapter 3 discusses the essential ingredients for a well-balanced, nutritious, and healthful diet.

When you find yourself under stress, you tend to eat whatever is available without thinking about its nutritional value. Foods rich in Vitamin B such as whole-grain cereals; sunflower, pumpkin or sesame seeds; eggs; and wheat germ or B complex vitamin pills are especially good. Your prenatal vitamins will usually include adequate doses of Vitamin B, but an additional increase in the total B complex helps to calm nerves. Since B vitamins are water soluble and any excess is washed out of the body via elimination, you do not have to worry about overdoing it. Increasing your intake of Vitamin C foods will also help to keep the body's defenses up. You should take no more than 1 gram (1000 mg.) of natural Vitamin C tablets. The "B's" and "C's" are the first vitamins to be burned up in times of stress or trauma.

Many minerals contribute to a feeling of good health, but iron deficiency can contribute to feelings of tiredness, anxiety, and fatigue. Be sure to have your iron levels checked if you experience any of these symptoms, for you may be suffering from pregnancy-induced anemia.

Conscious Breathing: The Key to Relaxation

You would think that, for all the ups and downs and mood swings of pregnancy, you would have to learn hundreds of techniques to become calm and centered. However, your body has its own set of controls that you can learn to use easily and effectively to reduce your stress levels. What is this secret mechanism that you possess? It's your breath!

Focusing all your attention on your child and on your body's natural breathing process for only a few minutes a day will produce amazing results. After introducing my students to abdominal or "Rock the Baby" breathing in their first PPF class, I usually instruct the women to try the breathing at red lights, while waiting in line at the supermarket, during television commercials. It is always fun to hear their success stories during the second class.

What is the deep dark secret behind this kind of breathing? It involves using the tummy or baby area while deep breathing, and total concentration on each breath. Sound simple? Not really. When I first describe abdominal breathing, one or two women always say that this technique is the opposite of the way they normally breathe. This may be true. However, it is much easier to learn abdominal breathing during pregnancy because of the added advantage of a prominent tummy.

This chapter contains a variety of breathing exercises that will naturally ease you over some of the rough spots and move you very smoothly into motherhood. Try all the breathing techniques at least once to see which ones you prefer. Check the varying benefits, so that you will know when to use each breath.

When you are practicing, you should really learn to focus both inward and outward. Focusing inward on the breathing pattern will help you to develop a slow, easy breathing rhythm. Focusing outward will help build your concentration skills. A geometric pattern has been provided below (see Figure 2.1) which you can use for outward concentration. Some women prefer inward concentration during labor, while others prefer outward concentration. You will have to tune into your own reactions during your labor experience. By spending some time each day or every other day on breathing exercises—even if you have never even heard of them until now—you will be in rhythm with your unborn baby. In addition, you will be practicing stress management skills.

The Physiology of Breathing

In order to take a really deep breath, you have to learn how to relax and use your abdominal muscles. Breathing with a tight tummy shrinks your body's air capacity, thereby allowing your diaphragm and rib muscles to grow weak while leaving the blood hungry for oxygen. Breathing in this way also puts more stress on the body; you have to take two or three shallow breaths to equal the amount of oxygen taken in with one deep abdominal breath.

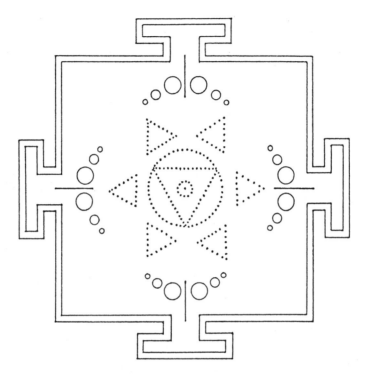

Figure 2.1　Mandala for Practicing Breathing Exercises

Some basic knowledge of your body's physiology will help you to understand the different processes involved when you take an abdominal breath. The parts of your body that are most directly involved in the breathing process are the nose (through which air travels), the trachea or windpipe (the connecting link to the lungs), and the lungs (where oxygen is exchanged for carbon dioxide with each breath). The heart and lungs are located in the thorax (chest cavity). The diaphragm (a thick muscle) forms the floor of the thorax. Below the thorax and the diaphragm is the abdominal area of your body, which contains the organs of digestion, reproduction, and excretion (see Figure 2.2). When you consciously relax the abdominal muscles and inhale, the diaphragm moves downward, thereby increasing your lung capacity (see Figure 2.3). At the same time, there is a reduction of air pressure in the lungs, and fresh air is forced into the lungs because of a vacuum-like pull. With the diaphramatic downstroke, the interior organs of the abdomen receive a gentle massage, which helps improve digestion and circulation. When exhaling, you have to slightly contract the abdominal wall. This will cause the diaphragm to return to a domed position pushing upward, and will expel carbon dioxide from your lungs (see Figure 2.4).

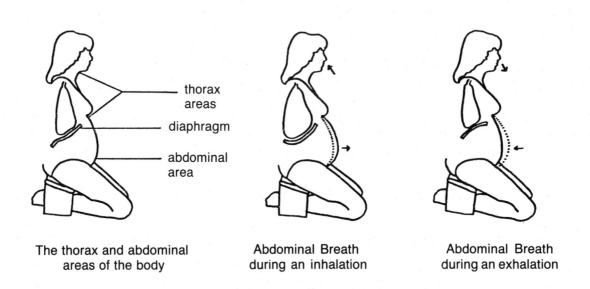

The thorax and abdominal areas of the body

Abdominal Breath during an inhalation

Abdominal Breath during an exhalation

Figures 2.2, 2.3, 2.4   PPF Abdominal Breathing Sequence

Shallow Breathing

Poor breathing habits can have a very negative effect on your body. Shallow (or upper chest) breathing usually leads to illness and can be accompanied by mental depression. As you carry and nurture your unborn child, you must be aware of how you can best fulfill the needs of this new person. Learning to breathe abdominally and avoiding shallow breathing can be one of the most positive steps you can take to insure your own well-being and that of your baby. Just as you are eating for two while you are pregnant, you are also breathing for two.

Breathing and Your Emotions

Have you ever noticed, in times of high emotion and sadness, that your breathing is very ragged and uneven? When you feel depressed, you may unconsciously lower your head and let your shoulders sag, thereby lessening your lung capacity. The more you cut down your lung capacity, however, the more depressed you will feel. The brain needs three times more oxygen than the rest of the body. No wonder you often make very little sense when you are highly emotional and upset! At such times, it is important to remember that the full responsibility for your emotional state is in your hands, or "lungs."

Guidelines for Practicing Breathing

The idea of "practicing breathing" may seem very strange to you, since you have been doing it all your life without any guidelines. However, in order to derive the most benefit from the following exercises, certain rules should be followed.

1. Check with your caregiver—either doctor or midwife—before beginning any breathing exercise program.

2. Use your nose for inhaling and exhaling, unless otherwise instructed. The nasal passages will clean, warm, and moisten the air before it enters your lungs and blood system.

3. *Never* hold your breath during these breathing exercises. This is bad for the baby.

4. Continually focus on either your body and baby or on the geometric pattern (see Figure 2.1) as you practice.

5. Practice each breath at least 5-10 times to achieve the desired results. It is the repetition and coordinated mental concentration that will cause you to either revitalize or calm down.

Abdominal Breath or "Rock the Baby" Breath

Benefits

- Consciously connects you to your future child.
- Calms your nerves.
- Increased oxygen intake enriches and purifies your blood and that of the baby's.
- Increases resistance to colds and other respiratory conditions.
- Can be used in the early stages of labor and at the beginning and end of each contraction in the later stages of labor.

Directions

1. Sitting in a cross-legged position on your mat, on a seiza bench, or comfortably in a chair, place your hands on your abdomen. Check to see that your head is up, your facial muscles are relaxed, and your back is as straight as possible (see Figure 2.5).

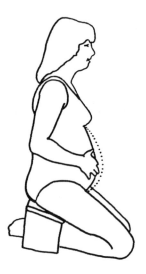

Figure 2.5 "Rock the Baby" Breath

2. Relax your tummy muscles and begin to inhale through your nose, sending the air directly to the baby area. Feel your abdomen move forward with the inhalation. Your shoulders, however, should be perfectly still.

3. Once you have completely filled your tummy area with air (this should take about five seconds), begin to smoothly exhale. *Do not hold your breath.*

4. As you exhale, which should take about 5-8 seconds, contract the abdomen, hugging your baby until the exhalation is complete. Notice that the tummy moves forward as you inhale and backward as you exhale. Hence the name "Rock the Baby" breath.

5. Be aware of your breath coming in and rocking your baby forward and your breath going out and rocking the baby backward. You may find that you concentrate better with your eyes closed.

6. Repeat 5-10 times and relax.

Cautions and Comments

- Do not practice this breath too fast or you may feel dizzy. Slowing down will cause any dizziness to disappear.
- With practice, you will find that you can inhale and exhale for longer periods of time. However, during the last six weeks of pregnancy, taking a deep breath will be more difficult and will take all your concentration and control.
- Do not rock your pelvis.
- Your baby may kick in appreciation for the extra boost of energy you are giving him when you practice this exercise. This is no cause for alarm.
- Once you have mastered this breath, you no longer have to keep your hands on your tummy.
- Practice this exercise at red lights, while waiting to see your caregiver, during television commercials—whenever you have a spare moment.
- In times of frenzy or uncertainty, this breath will calm you.

Alternate Nostril Breath (or The Headache Remedy)

Benefits

- Calms both your body and your mind.
- Helps you to overcome such negative feelings as fear, worry, and anxiety.
- Helps to relieve sinus conditions.
- Strengthens your nervous system.
- Can minimize and/or eliminate headaches and insomnia.
- Can help to keep blood pressure at normal levels.
- Makes you feel very peaceful and serene.

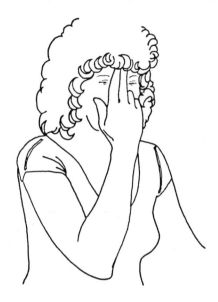

Figure 2.6 Alternate Nostril Breath

Directions

1. Sitting cross-legged on your mat or in a comfortable chair (with your back and head up straight), bring your right palm up in front of your face.

2. Bend the fourth and fifth fingers of your right hand. Lightly block the left nostril with these fingers. Leave your right nostril open (see Figure 2.6).

3. Relax your facial muscles and close your eyes. Begin inhaling smoothly and evenly with the right nostril, using "Rock the Baby" breath. When you have inhaled as fully as you can (without straining), close it off with your thumb.

4. Open the left nostril by moving your fourth finger and exhaling completely on the left side (see Figure 2.7). The exhalation will usually be longer than the inhalation. Once the exhalation is complete, close off the left side again

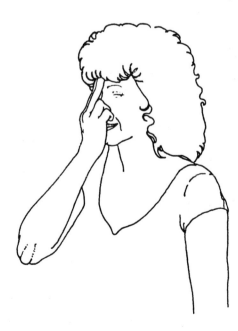

Figure 2.7 Alternate Nostril Breath

and begin to inhale with the right. Repeat this same procedure for five breaths. (Breathe in right and out left, five times.)

5. After the fifth breath, change the sequence by inhaling with the left and exhaling with the right for five breaths.

6. After completing ten rounds of breaths, rest your hands in your lap, keep your eyes closed, and relax for a while.

Cautions and Comments

•Breathe evenly, quietly, and without strain even though one nostril may be more open than the other. If you feel you are not inhaling enough, use your mouth for part of the inhalation. Exhale through your nose.

•If you have a stuffed nose, you might try inhaling completely through the mouth and exhaling completely through the nose. These movements will help to temporarily clear out stuffed noses.

•Follow the breath mentally with each inhalation and exhalation.

•If you feel a headache coming on, this is an excellent remedy.

•This breath (which is derived from yoga) is often called the sun/moon breath, since it is believed that one nostril is active and positive (sun) while the other is passive and negative (moon). Alternate nostril breathing restores equilibrium by balancing the opposite currents of the body.

•Practice this breath for ten rounds before practicing relaxation.

Anti-Insomnia Breath

Benefits

•Helps to eliminate insomnia.
•Strengthens your breathing mechanism.
•Slows down your body systems and your brain without the use of harmful drugs.
•Develops your concentration skills.

Directions

1. Lying on your left side in a comfortable position, lightly close off your right nostril with your right thumb.

2. Close your eyes. Inhale and exhale with only the left nostril, using "Rock the Baby" breath.

3. Do 15 smooth, slow inhalations and 15 even, complete exhalations.

4. It is very important to concentrate on counting your breaths (this helps to put you to sleep!).

5. When you have finished breathing, get comfortable and begin a complete mental relaxation (see page 158).

6. Begin by relaxing your facial muscles, then your neck, etc.

7. Let yourself fall off to sleep.

Cautions and Comments

- If you can't get back to sleep in the middle of the night, it is often useful to drink a hot glass of milk, read for 10-15 minutes, then go back to bed and practice this breath.
- If you are left-handed, these directions should be reversed. For left-handed people, the passive or sleep-inducing nostril is the right one. *Remember that your dominant or active nostril is the same as your dominant hand. Only using the dominant or active nostril for breathing will energize you. Only using the passive nostril will put you to sleep.*

Baby Breath

Benefits

- Mentally and physically prepares you to utilize the birth canal in your baby's birth.
- Reminds you of the birth process on a daily basis.
- Helps to keep your sexual muscles well toned.
- Calms your nerves.
- Energizes and revitalizes your entire being.

Directions

1. Stand up straight on your mat, with your feet 8-10 inches apart.

2. Turn your feet outward at a 45° angle. Stretch your arms out straight in front of your chest, palms down.

3. Slowly go down into a regular squatting position (see Figure 2.8) standing either on your toes or on flat feet. You may want to have a chair in front of you for support, if you have not yet mastered squatting.

4. Once you are in a squatting position, rest your hands on your knees or clasp them in front of you.

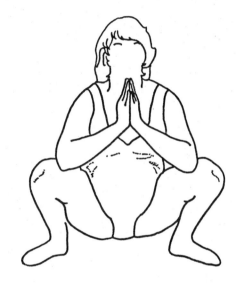

Figure 2.8 A Squatting Position for Practicing "Baby Breath"

5. Relax all of your facial muscles. As you begin to inhale, *imagine* that you are inhaling through your navel directly to the baby. Your tummy will move slightly forward.

6. As you exhale *imagine* that you are exhaling through the birth canal as you push down and forward slightly, using your vaginal muscles. *Imagine* that the breath is taking the same route that your baby will take at the time of birth.

7. Feel the bottom of your tummy contracting as you exhale.

8. Repeat five times and relax.

Cautions and Comments

- Do not be discouraged if it takes you awhile to learn this breath. The effort will surely be worth it!
- Do not push down too hard—it is a very subtle movement.

- One student commented on this breath: "My doctor and nurses were amazed at how well I was able to push. I really feel that the idea of 'Baby Breath' (exhaling through the birth canal) made this part of delivery easy."
- Practicing this breath will help to facilitate and possibly even shorten your pushing time when you are in labor.
- Practice this breath between exercises, while driving, etc.

Energizing Single Nostril Breath

Benefits

- Energizes your body and mind.
- Increases alertness while eliminating fatigue.
- Strengthens your breathing mechanism.
- Improves your concentration skills.

Directions

1. Arrange yourself in any comfortable position.

2. Close off your left nostril with your right pointer finger.

3. Close your eyes. Inhale and exhale with the right nostril using only the "Rock the Baby" breath. Do 10 smooth, slow inhalations and 10 even, complete exhalations.

4. As you inhale, think, "Inhale energy one." As you exhale, think, "Exhale tiredness one;" then continue, "In-hale energy two," "Exhale tiredness two," etc., until you reach ten. It is very important to keep your mental concentration on these thoughts, for you are reprogramming your body.

5. Relax the right hand and keep your eyes closed as your breathing returns to normal upon completion of the ten rounds.

6. Within 5-10 minutes you will begin to feel revitalized and renewed.

Cautions and Comments

- Do not substitute this breath for sleep when your body is truly tired.
- If you are left-handed, these directions should be reversed. For left-handed people, the dominant nostril is the left one.

Sighing Breath

Benefits

- Releases stored tensions, anxieties, hidden thoughts and fears.
- Flushes the lungs of wastes.
- Refreshes and recharges the body.
- Helps break down conditioning against making sounds.

Directions

1. Arrange yourself in any comfortable position. Relax your facial muscles and close your eyes.

2. Inhale fully and smoothly using "Rock the Baby" breath.

3. Exhale through your mouth, allowing the air to touch the back of your throat. It should sound like a soft sighing "haa" sound.

4. When you are practicing this breath, imagine that you have just finished an unenjoyable chore and are sighing with relief now that it is over.

5. Repeat 5-10 times and rest.

Cautions and Comments

- Do not force the air out; merely let it come out naturally.
- Be dramatic when you sigh. If you are, many stored-up tensions will disappear.
- This breath will teach you that it is all right to make some sounds during labor. Do not be embarrassed. Sounds can enhance the progress of labor by quickly letting go of the tensions accumulated during a contraction. It is wise to end every contraction with one or two soft Sighing Breaths. In essence you are expressing your relief that the contraction is over.

Smooth Breath

Benefits

- Quiets, calms, relaxes, and stabilizes the mind and body.
- Develops excellent control of the breathing process.
- Helps to ensure emotional balance.
- Helps to develop your concentration skills.

Directions

1. Arrange yourself in any comfortable position. Relax your facial muscles.

2. Focusing all your attention on your breathing, begin to inhale using "Rock the Baby" breath. Make the inhalation as smooth as possible. Imag-

ine that your breath is beginning to surround your sleeping baby.

3. As you begin to exhale, imagine the breath completing its circle around the baby and coming back up to your nose for exhalation.

4. Make sure that the change from inhalation to exhalation is as quiet and smooth as possible, so as not to disturb the baby. Allow your breath to caress and energize your baby, but do not wake it up!

5. Practice 5-10 breaths and then rest.

Cautions and Comments

•This breath may seem difficult at first, but with practice it will become very enjoyable.

•The control learned by practicing this breath will be very helpful to you during labor.

•Try not to pause between inhalations and exhalations. Make the transition as smooth as you can.

CHAPTER THREE
Nutrition In Pregnancy

Look at the French word "la nourriture." Can you see a similarity to an English word? If you noticed a resemblance to the English verb "to nourish," you were right. "La nourriture" is the French word for food, and it reflects a basic understanding of one of the most important values of eating. The foods you eat should satisfy your tastes and desires while nourishing, developing, and sustaining both your body and your baby's body, brain, and being. During pregnancy you can begin to educate yourself about balanced eating in preparation for feeding your child in the coming years. In addition, by cultivating good nutritional habits, you can avoid many of the uncomfortable side effects of pregnancy. Recent research has indicated a definite link between proper nutrition, elimination of negative pregnancy experiences, and a healthy baby. Only recently has it become clear that all foods that are eaten can and do affect the growing baby. The varied and well-balanced diet which is recommended within this chapter will be useful to you while you are expecting, while you are breastfeeding, and eventually for good health and vitality during your entire life. The diet is based on recommendations stated in the California Department of Health's report, *Nutrition During Pregnancy and Lactation* (1975), as well as on consultations with clinical dieticians.

THE PPF APPROACH TO FOOD

There are some simple rules which should be considered in your choice, preparation, and consumption of food:

1. Eat a large variety of foods from the four basic food groups: proteins, calcium sources, whole grains and starchy products, and fresh fruits and vegetables. This variety of foods will provide all the essentials necessary for your body to maintain itself and build a baby. The balance should increase your knowledge of nutrition, as well as contribute to good health.

2. Eat slowly and chew your food well. The digestion process begins in the mouth. Since stomach space becomes limited as the pregnancy progresses, chewing well will ensure smoother digestion.

3. Eat foods as close to their natural state as possible. Try eating some raw foods daily. Foods in their natural state contain the energy of life. Foods which are denatured by refining, preserving, canning, smoking, etc., lose this vital energy and are often "dead food." Choose fresh foods first, frozen foods second, and canned foods last.

4. When using processed foods, read the labels carefully to see what you and your baby are eating. If you can't pronounce it, do you really want to eat it? Many food additives have not been adequately tested, especially in relationship to cancer and birth defects. Why take chances? Additives to avoid are nitrites and nitrates; artificial colors and flavors; BHA and BHT; saccharin and cyclamates.

5. Cook your vegetables for a minimal time. Using a perforated steamer is best. You will retain the most vitamins and minerals by quick cooking. When vegetables are cooked this way, they are brightly colored and extremely appealing to the eye. Use the water which is left in the bottom of the vegetable cooking pan as a highly-nutritious, low-calorie chilled drink or as a base for soups.

6. Eat five to six small meals a day. (Don't eat more; eat more often.) Eating smaller amounts will keep your energy levels stable. When you are famished, you are more likely to reach for a candy bar than a salad. Eating small, high-protein meals lessens the burden on your stomach and diminishes the likelihood of nausea and/or heartburn.

7. Eat only when your body feels hungry. Do not be pressured into eating when you are not really hungry. Do not feel that you need to conform to the usual standard times for meals. Learn to tune in to your body and detect when you are eating to fulfill hunger rather than eating to combat boredom or to be sociable.

8. Have a positive attitude toward the food you are eating. Close your eyes as you eat and really taste your food. Notice the texture of the food as well. Think of your food as the building blocks of your own and your baby's health and development. Enjoy your food by really paying attention to how it tastes.

9. Do not eat when you are under emotional stress or are extremely tired. Wait until you have calmed down (do some "Rock the Baby" breathing) or until after you have taken a nap. Your body may have difficulty digesting the food if you are in a heightened or depressed state. This is why indigestion usually goes hand-in-hand with emotional upsets.

Following these simple and logical rules will help to improve your eating habits, while ensuring more enjoyment from your meals.

HOW THE BODY WORKS

At one time or another during this pregnancy, you may have marveled at the workings of nature. Your baby began as two single cells and may now be kicking even as you read this. The workings of the body are truly miraculous and complicated. In order to maintain the body while building a baby, you must consume the proper "building materials" each day.

Imagine that you are a worker in a vast factory and are trying to build a baby heart cell. You have to gather all the basic ingredients from which a baby heart cell is made. You come across an obstacle, however: one basic ingredient cannot be found. Your boss tells you to search all over to find the missing ingredient. You follow his orders and look everywhere. You look in the body's stored reserves. You check into the areas where the body manufactures cells. But that special ingredient cannot be found. "Well," says the boss, "I guess we can't do that job today. We'll have to wait until the missing ingredient comes in."

This is a very simplified imaginary story, but the main point is valid. If you are missing a basic ingredient, the cells in question cannot be manufactured. Although you may not want to know all about the inner workings of your body, it is extremely important to know which major ingredients have to be consumed each day to keep your body and your baby healthy.

Protein

Protein is used by the body to form the basic structure of every cell, as well as to build and maintain all the cells that compose the baby's body, the uterus, and the placenta. This nutrient plays a vital role in the production of brain cells in the growing fetus. Thus, adequate protein consumption is necessary for the future mental development of your child. Frequent high protein intake can eliminate the nausea of early pregnancy and prevent the toxemia which can develop in late pregnancy.

Many foods contain protein; however, there are complete and incomplete proteins. Women who are on vegetarian or other regulated diets during pregnancy must be very careful to fulfill their daily complete protein requirement. It is possible to form complete proteins by mixing two incomplete proteins in one meal. Reading and studying

Diet for a Small Planet by Frances Moore Lappe (Ballantine Books, revised edition, 1985), which contains thorough explanations on how to mix incomplete proteins in the correct proportions to form complete proteins, should be mandatory for women on restricted diets. If you are on a limited diet, it is very important for you to keep a food diary (see instructions on page 32) so that you will be sure to eat adequate amounts of protein. Also, vegetarian pregnant women should supplement their diets with B_{12} daily. Check with your doctor or midwife for amounts.

According to the Food and Nutrition Board of the National Academy of Sciences, the 1980 Recommended Daily Dietary Allowances (RDA) during pregnancy is a minimum of 74 grams of protein per day. Many nutritionists suggest 100 grams a day from the fifth month until the end of the pregnancy, to insure adequate brain development in the child as well as good health in the mother. A good pamphlet to read and study on prenatal nutrition is "As You Eat So Your Baby Grows" by Nikki Goldbeck, revised edition, 1986. (See the Bibliography for mailing address.)

Calcium

This nutrient is the main ingredient for forming healthy bones and teeth in your baby. Both calcium and phosphorous must be included in your daily diet, especially during the last three months of your pregnancy. If your calcium intake is not high enough, your body will use its own bone cells to supply the baby. A lack of calcium can cause muscle cramps (usually in the calves), sleeplessness, irritability, and increased tooth decay. Even if you do not like milk, you can fulfill your daily requirement by eating foods in the dairy group. If you are not drinking milk or eating other calcium food sources, you may want to talk to your doctor or midwife about supplementing your diet with calcium pills.

Vitamins

Vitamins are live substances within your food which play an important role in how well your body functions. Since they are live substances, they can be affected by heat, light, canning, freezing, and processing. That is why processed food products have to be vitamin-fortified. Fresh, raw foods contain high amounts of a wide variety of vitamins. However, if you allow your food to remain in the refrigerator for long periods of time, the vitamins deteriorate. The freezing and canning processes kill a high percentage of the vitamins in food. The vitamins found in oils, such as vitamins A, D, and E, are fat soluble and can be stored in the body. An oversupply of these vitamins can be toxic and have very serious and dangerous effects on your body. That is why supplemental vitamins must be taken with care and knowledge. The water soluble vitamins, such as the B complex (there are 11 recognized vitamins in this group) and C, cannot be stored and must be replenished daily. Otherwise, symptoms of deficiency result. Vitamin C is very perishable and is destroyed by extreme heat and contact with the air. It is wise to prepare Vitamin C rich foods right before you plan to eat them. If you are in a stressful situation, you will immediately burn up the B and C Vitamins present in your body. Smoking cigarettes severely depletes your Vitamin C supply. If you continue to smoke while pregnant (although you really should not), you should increase your daily intake of Vitamin C by increasing the number of fruits and vegetables high in Vitamin C in your diet. The RDA for Vitamin C is 80 mgs. daily for pregnant women.

Iron

Iron is an essential mineral which enables the hemoglobin (the red coloring matter in your blood) to carry oxygen to every cell of your body and the baby's. If your diet does not contain enough iron, you may develop anemia, fatigue, and shortness of breath. According to the Food and Nutrition Board of the National Academy of Sciences, the increased iron requirement cannot be met by the iron content of usual American diets or by the iron stores of many pregnant women. Therefore, an iron supplement of 30-60 mgs. daily should be taken. During the last three months of pregnancy, your baby's iron reserves are being formed; therefore, it is imperative to keep your iron intake high. The baby will be unable to utilize ingested iron very well in the first three months of its life, and so will use these reserves during that time. Foods which are high in iron are fresh fruits (especially apricots), green leafy vegetables, prune juice, almonds, liver, egg yolk, wheat germ, and blackstrap molasses.

If you are a vegetarian or do not care for liver, you can use cast-iron cooking utensils two to three times a day—for cooking your eggs in the morning, grilling a cheese sandwich at lunch, or cooking your evening vegetable. You should make sure that you eat Vitamin C rich foods, such as orange juice, with your eggs, or a tomato in the grilled cheese sandwich to boost iron absorption.

Almost all pregnant women take an iron supplement of 30-60 mgs. in pill form. You should be aware that there are a variety of supplements available. Often pregnant women find that they become very constipated from these supplements. Ferrous sulfate should not be taken during pregnancy because it destroys Vitamin E very quickly. Other kinds of iron supplements which have been found to be effective but not constipating are ferrous gluconate, ferrous fumurate (FemIron) or ferrous sulfate with molybdenum (MolIron). Iron supplementation should be continued all during the time you breastfeed or bottle-feed your baby.

Weight Gain

Most pregnant women are very concerned about the amount of weight they gain during the waiting months. A weight gain is a natural indicator that the body is changing and growing to facilitate the development of the baby. The dietary require-ments which have been recommended in this chapter are necessary to accommodate the increase in your body's metabolism and tissue production, as well as the growth of the baby. Weight gain during pregnancy should, therefore, be regarded as a positive aspect of the pregnancy. Your mental attitude about this change in your body shape will have a very definite effect on you, so you should spend some time sorting out your feelings.

Most doctors and midwives agree that a weight gain of 21-30 pounds is desirable for a healthy baby. During your prenatal checkups, you will be monitored very carefully, for there should be a definite pattern to this weight gain. During the first trimester there should be a very minimal weight gain of two to four lbs. During the second trimester, when much growth takes place, you should gain about three to four lbs. a month. During the last trimester your weight gain will reflect the baby putting on weight in preparation for birth. You should not limit your diet, especially during the last trimester, for it will directly deprive your baby of good birth weight and a chance for good health.

VEGETARIAN DIETS AND PREGNANCY

Yoga and vegetarian eating seem to be naturally linked in this country. However, in order to thrive on a vegetarian diet, you must have a basic knowledge of nutrition and complementary proteins. This takes some study and understanding. People often become vegetarians without this prior knowledge, and the results are disastrous, such as a lack of energy, irritability, and illness.

If you do plan to follow a vegetarian diet during pregnancy, you should consider the diet Gail Sforza Brewer has detailed in *The Brewer Medical Diet for Normal and High-Risk Pregnancy* (see the Appendix). Ms. Brewer has researched vegetarian diets for lacto-ovo and vegan vegetarians and has developed two separate comprehensive diets. By following the diet recommended in this book, you can be sure that your baby thrives while meeting your own nutritional requirements.

FOOD DIARY

Use a food diary as your guide for evaluating your diet. Write down in a notebook or on a sheet of paper what you eat throughout the day. Include breakfast, lunch, and supper, as well as mid-morning, afternoon, and evening snacks. Does your daily diet contain the prescribed number of servings from each food group? Is it varied? Are you eating 4-6 small meals a day? Are you eating only when hungry?

HERBS AND PREGNANCY

The use of natural remedies has been growing in popularity during the past few years. Many people are turning to herbal remedies because they prefer a more natural approach. With the relationship between increased stress and caffeine consumption

CHECKLIST FOR DAILY FOOD DIARY DURING PREGNANCY

Remember to eat the correct amount daily from each food group.

		Servings Per Day:

Group I	Complete protein
	  Meat
	  Meatless
	  Complementary
		2-3 3 oz. servings

Group II	Calcium sources	Four servings (1 serving = 8 oz. of milk or the equivalent)
Group III	Whole grain products and starchy vegetables	Four servings (1 serving = 1 slice of bread or its equivalent)
Group IV	Fruits and vegetables with Vitamin C Leafy green vegetables with Vitamin A, folic acid and iron Other fruits and vegetables with Vitamin A	One serving (1 serving = 1 orange or its equivalent) Two servings (1 serving = 1 cup or its equivalent) One serving ($1/2$ cup or its equivalent)
Others	Butter; vegetable oil; fortified margarine; salt to taste Liquids Snacks (Dried fruits, unsalted nuts, sunflower seeds, unsalted popcorn)	One to two tablespoons Six to eight glasses a day One to three daily

being more clearly understood and accepted, more people are turning to caffeine-free herbal teas. From a PPF point of view, herbal teas can be most beneficial if you learn some basic information about the herbs that you are drinking. You must remember that herbs are a form of medicine and that some herbs can have a very negative effect on your body.

Herb teas should be prepared only in glass, porcelain, ceramic or enamel cups and pots. They should never touch metal in their preparation. Boiling water should be poured over the herbs (fresh or dried), steeped for 3-5 minutes, then strained with a bamboo strainer before drinking. Most teas are pleasant-tasting, especially when they are made properly. Herbal teas will not become as dark as English, Indian, or Chinese teas. For sweetness, you can add a bit of honey or a squeeze of lemon.

Red Raspberry Leaf Tea

Historically, Red Raspberry leaf tea, or Rubus Ideaus (see Figure 3.1) has been known as the best and most helpful herbal tea for pregnancy, birth, and lactation. Red Raspberry leaves have a very beneficial effect on the female reproductive organs. Additionally, they have a soothing effect on nausea, prevent miscarriage, ease labor pains, and build up a healthy milk supply. Many women who have consumed this tea during labor and after the baby's birth have reported an easier and less painful birthing experience and a reduction in afterbirth cramps.

According to Nan Ullrike Koehler, author of *Artemis Speaks: With VBAC Stories and Natural Childbirth Information* (Jerry Brown, 1985), herbs have four basic functions:

1. Most importantly, they are a source of minerals. Red Raspberry leaf tea is an excellent source of calcium and magnesium. It has a relaxing effect on the muscles and nerves. It is considered a uterine tonic and may contribute to Braxton-Hicks contractions throughout pregnancy. These practice contractions prepare the uterus and cervix for the rigors of birth.

2. Plant alkaloids (the medicinally-active components) are released when boiling water bursts the plant cell walls. It isn't known exactly how Red Raspberry leaf works on the uterus, except that it is a good source of minerals and has mild astringent properties. Empirical evidence suggests that it acts on muscle tissues and promotes general health as an antiacid and blood purifier through the calcium, magnesium, and iron that it seems to concentrate.

3. The physical effort of preparing a cup of tea is a positive step toward a good birth. You should take the time to fix 1-4 cups of tea daily, focusing inward for the moment on the new life that you will soon bring into the world.

4. It is important to obtain adequate fluids all through the pregnancy and to avoid dehydration. Begin drinking one cup of Red Raspberry leaf tea daily early in pregnancy. In the last 3-4 weeks, you should drink four cups a day. In the last month of pregnancy, you might also add Black Cohosh, Blessed Thistle, Squaw Vine, and Pennyroyal to the Red Raspberry leaves, all in a 1:1 ratio. These stimulate and nourish the uterus so that, by the time you are in labor, most of the work is already done. If you can remain well hydrated (this means drinking 3-4 quarts of water per day), most of the unpleasant symptoms of pregnancy and labor difficulties will be eliminated.

Red Raspberry leaf tea has a mild flavor and is available in most health food stores or through PPF (see the Appendix). It is very nice hot or cold. You should not exceed four cups a day, however, in late pregnancy—this may cause preterm labor.

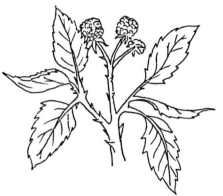

Figure 3.1 Red Raspberry Leaf Tea
(Rubus Ideaus)

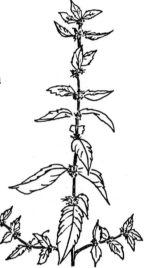

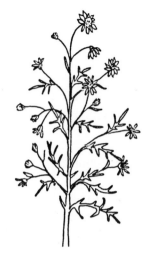

Figure 3.3 Camomile
(Matricaria or Anthemis Nobilis)

Figure 3.2 Peppermint
(Mentha Piperita)

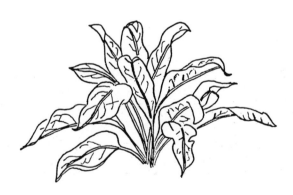

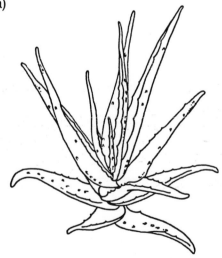

Figure 3.4 Comfrey
(Symphytum Officinale)

Figure 3.5 Aloe Vera

GETTING RELIEF FROM HERBS

Nausea

Peppermint tea (Mentha piperita) is helpful for eliminating nausea or an upset stomach. Warm tea is often more helpful than cold (see Figure 3.2). *Camomile* tea (Matricaria or anthemis nobilis) relieves many ailments, especially those in the womb and stomach. It helps to eliminate vomiting if consumed in the morning. It has been known to relieve intestinal gas as well.

Sleeplessness

Camomile is very soothing when drunk while still hot, with a bit of honey if you prefer. Celestial Seasonings Herb Tea Co. produces a mixture called "Sleepytime," which contains camomile and other assorted herbs. This is a very soothing and often sleep-inducing, safe tea for pregnancy (see Figure 3.3).

Postpartum Healing

Comfrey tea (Symphytum officinale) is exceedingly helpful for healing wounds. Crushing a fresh leaf to release the juices and placing it over your sanitary pad will help to heal up the episiotomy or other tears. If you prefer, you can make a tea from three teaspoons of comfrey leaf and one cup of hot water, simmered for 20 minutes. After straining and cooling the tea, a soft cloth can be dipped into the warm tea and applied to the wound area to promote healing (see Figure 3.4).

Birthing

As already mentioned, *Red Raspberry* (Rubus Ideaus) is known to promote a relaxed delivery and is an astringent.

Spikenard tea (Aralia racemosa) is known as a blood purifier and is recommended during the last six weeks of pregnancy in combination with Red Raspberry leaf.

Cracked Nipples

Aloe Vera is good for cracked nipples. Try cutting a piece of the Aloe Vera plant and applying the moist part to the damaged nipple. Repeat a few minutes later after the nipple has dried. At the next feeding, you should use the other breast only. Before you use the treated nipple, wash it carefully with warm water. Repeat the Aloe Vera application after each feeding until the nipple has healed (see Figure 3.5).

HERBS TO WATCH OUT FOR

Before using any substance, you should be aware of its effects on your body. The following herbs can have very negative effects if used in the wrong proportion or at the wrong time. Unless you are working with a trained herbologist, you should avoid the following substances during pregnancy and lactation.

Lobelia (Lobelia inflata) is a very strong herb which can act as both a stimulant and a relaxant. Excessive dosages can induce continual vomiting. *Peach tree leaves* must be used in specific quantities because the leaves and flowers contain small amounts of hydrocyanic acid, which is poisonous. Excess use of these leaves can cause diarrhea. *Blue Cohosh* is often irritating to the mucous membranes, but it has been used by women to strengthen their uterine contractions during labor. Other herbal teas to avoid are *Golden Seal, Yarrow, Valerian, Tansy, Cotton Root, Motherwort, Couchgrass, Rue, Vervain* and *St. John's Wort.* These teas can begin uterine contractions and thus cause a miscarriage.

You may want to check the bibliography for a listing of books on herbs so that you can become more familiar with their properties and benefits. Always check the ingredients when buying herbal teas to see that they do not contain the above-mentioned detrimental herbs. New herbal teas known as "pregnancy brews" are available at some health food stores. If you buy a "pregnancy tea," it should contain Red Raspberry leaf in combination with two or three other herbs. Experimenting with the different tastes which herbal teas can provide can be a new and interesting aspect of your pregnancy.

CAUTIONS AND COMMENTS FOR PREGNANCY NUTRITION

- Do not take diuretics (water pills), which can flush important minerals out of your system.
- Do not use any antihistamines to unclog a stuffy nose. Instead, fill an empty spray bottle with warm water and spray this into your nose to relieve congestion.
- Do not take antacids or laxatives without your caregiver's consent.
- Do not take motion sickness or anti-nausea (Bendictin) medications because they have been linked with birth defects.
- Do not take steroids and herbs containing steroid-like properties including agave, ginseng, licorice, hops, and sage.
- Minimize your consumption of caffeine foods such as coffee, leaf tea, cola drinks, and cocoa. The connection between high caffeine intake and birth defects is now being researched. Drink herbal teas, grain coffee substitutes like Postum and Pero, unsweetened fruit juices, mineral water or iced water with half a lemon squeezed into it.
- Do not diet during pregnancy even if you were overweight when you became pregnant. This may cause birth defects in your future child.

- Do not fast during pregnancy. Going without food for even 24 hours is not good for your growing baby.
- Do not smoke. If you must, cut down to only a few cigarettes daily. The smoke in your system deprives your unborn child of necessary oxygen. Babies with low birth weight or premature babies are often born to mothers who smoke. Pregnant women who smoke should increase their Vitamin C intake.
- Do not take chemical stimulants and depressants such as LSD, marijuana, phenobarbital, psychotropics, barbiturates, or tranquilizers.
- Alcohol, consumed even in moderate amounts, may cause birth defects in your child. It may also cause physical and behavioral abnormalities. If you want to aid in your baby's healthy development, drink non-alcoholic beverages such as Perrier water with lemon or cranberry juice with lime at social functions.
- Try to keep your intake of chemical additives at a minimum. Luncheon meats contain nitrates and nitrites, so substitute sliced home-cooked turkey, chicken, chopped liver or roast beef.
- Drink 6-8 glasses of liquid daily in the form of water, unsweetened fruit juices, herbal teas, grain coffee substitutes, vegetable juices, etc.
- Salt your food according to taste. If swelling occurs in your legs, you should talk to your caregiver about resting with the legs higher than your heart. Do not completely eliminate salt from your diet, as it is necessary for proper body metabolism.
- Avoid raw or undercooked meat and fish.
- Do not expose yourself to radiation in the form of X-rays or video display terminals.
- Avoid contact with paints, thinners, solvents, wood preservatives, varnishes, benzene, dry-cleaning fluids, glues, spray adhesives, and vinyl chloride.
- Avoid hair dyes.
- Snack often during the day, choosing foods that are nutritious as well as tasty.
- Try to keep your white sugar consumption at a minimum. Use honey or molasses instead, but sparingly. Sugar contributes to increased tooth decay, as well as emotional ups and downs.
- Keep a food diary for several days each month so that you will be able to check your diet. You should be eating foods from the four basic food groups. Using a food diary is an easy way to learn all the fundamentals of good nutrition.
- Avoid greasy fried foods, fats, and gravies.
- Above all, have a *positive mental attitude* as you nourish and build your happy and healthy new baby.

CHAPTER FOUR

Natural Aids for Some Common Pregnancy Complaints

The experience of pregnancy is as varied as the babies that arrive when the pregnancy culminates. The variety of pregnancy complaints covers a wide scope. Some of these complaints are very subtle and disappear very quickly, while others may linger for months and sometimes last throughout the entire pregnancy. Since medication of any sort is usually forbidden during pregnancy, natural remedies which can eliminate or minimize the problem are most useful.

This chapter will discuss some of pregnancy's most common complaints and some natural remedies using PPF physical exercises, dietary changes, breathing, cleansing and relaxing techniques, as well as general information to relieve a worried mind. It is very important to remember that any dietary supplement such as vitamins must be approved by your doctor or midwife. *Do not take any pills without your doctor's or midwife's consent*.

Although all the information in this chapter will be useful, your situation may be different from the general situation which has been described. Dosages of vitamins vary according to your specific situation. After you have obtained your doctor's or midwife's approval for using the exercises and dietary changes, keep them well informed about your progress in alleviating the complaint. You will notice that many of the most common pregnancy complaints are due to inadequate or improperly balanced nutritional patterns. By keeping track of what you are eating via a food diary, you will be sure to know whether your diet is nutritionally sufficient for both you and the baby.

Backache

Useful Exercises

- Good posture (p.69)
- Alternate Leg Stretch to the side (p.119)
- Bridge (p. 81)
- Hip Rotator (p. 106)
- Lower Back Rocker (p. 83)
- Pelvic Circles (p. 80)
- Pendulum Legs (p. 115)
- Spinal Twist (p. 76)
- Salute to the Child (p. 94)
- Universal Pose (p. 116)

Cautions and Comments

- Do not do any forward bending or strong upward stretching exercises.
- Do not wear high-heeled shoes; they increase the likelihood of backache.
- Do not stay in one position for long periods of time.

Tips and Other Information

- Learn to take 2-3 minute stretch periods during the day.
- Soak a small towel in Cider Vinegar. Squeeze off the excess vinegar. Lay down in bed on your side and spread the towel directly across your back. Enjoy talking to your baby as the cool, delicious feeling pervades your body. Relax for 15-30 minutes and watch your backache disappear.

Bleeding Gums

Useful Exercises

- Floss your teeth daily or use a water pick.
- Brush your teeth and gums 3-4 times a day. Rinse your mouth well.
- Massage gums with your fingers when necessary. Be sure your hands are clean.

Cautions and Comments

- Be sure your diet contains enough calcium and high-quality, complete proteins.
- A Vitamin C deficiency can contribute to bleeding gums. Increase your intake of Vitamin C rich foods.

•Smoking will cause Vitamin C to be negated, so if you smoke, either cut down or quit altogether.

•See your dentist at least once during your pregnancy.

•*Do not* have any X-rays taken at this time.

Tips and Other Information

•Keep in mind that gum problems are most severe during the last weeks of pregnancy.

Constipation

Useful Exercises

•Knee-to-Chest position (on side): Lie on your side. Bend top knee and place it near your chest. Wrap your arm around your knee and hold, breathing normally for 15-20 seconds. Keep your head on a mat throughout. Repeat on the other side. Do this exercise 2-5 times.

•"Rock the Baby" breath will stimulate the intestinal area. Do ten breaths (p. 19).

Cautions and Comments

•Add fresh and dried fruits (prunes, raisins, figs, etc.) to your daily diet.

•Eat fresh vegetables and salads containing a variety of raw green and colored vegetables daily.

•Drink 6-8 glasses of liquid (including water) each day.

•Eat whole grain breads, cereals, and whole bran flakes. Begin with two teaspoons of bran in a glass of apple juice twice a day. The bran may cause some gas until your system gets used to it.

•Do not take bottled laxatives without your doctor's or midwife's approval.

Tips and Other Information

•Increasing progesterone in your system makes the bowels less efficient.

•Walking a mile a day is very helpful.

•Set a regular time each day to move your bowels.

•Keeping your feet and legs elevated on a footstool during elimination helps to move the bowels by releasing the anal muscles.

•An enema using body temperature water may be used occasionally if all else fails.

Dizziness

Useful Exercises

- Practicing all exercises at a slow pace will train you to move slowly and avoid this problem.
- Slow, deep abdominal breathing ("Rock the Baby" breath) with your legs elevated on a 45° angle

Cautions and Comments

- Do not change positions quickly. Take your time and focus on what you are doing.

Tips and Other Information

- Your blood pressure may drop due to the pressure of your uterus on major blood vessels, thus causing dizziness.

Gas (Flatulence)

Useful Exercises

- Zen sitting position for five minutes after meals helps digestion (p. 102)
- Squatting postures, if you do not have varicose veins (p. 97)
- Knees on chest and rock, if comfortable (p. 83)
- Knee to chest, on side (p. 84)

Cautions and Comments

- Eat 4-5 small meals a day.
- Chew your food slowly and well.
- Avoid foods which cause you to have gas. Keeping a food diary will enable you to find out this information.
- Cook your foods quickly using a perforated steamer, instead of boiling for long periods of time.
- To reduce gas-causing sulphur compounds in beans (including pinto, garbanzo, navy, etc.), bring one cup of beans to a boil in five cups of water. Boil for one minute. Drain and add five fresh cups of water. Bring to a second boil and cook according to directions.
- Gas may be a result of eating certain foods together. Keeping a food diary will help you to discover unfavorable food combinations.

Tips and Other Information

- Walking one mile a day should help digestion and elimination.
- Setting a regular time to move your bowels will be helpful.

Groin Spasm, Stitch, or Pressure

Useful Exercises

- Half Bow on Side (p. 85)
- Half Bow Standing (p. 113)
- Salute to the Child, #7 and #8 (p. 94)
- Squatting positions
- Knee to Chest, on side (p. 84)
- Pregnancy Triangle (p. 108). Do this with both legs straight.
- Alternate Leg Stretch to the side (p. 119)

Cautions and Comments

- Breathe deeply during the spasm. Bend toward the point of pain, thereby allowing the ligament to relax. Relax in a side-lying position until the spasm is over (p. 157).
- Only practice the PPF exercises that don't aggravate this area.

Tips and Other Information

- This is often felt as a stitch on the right side. The round ligaments connecting the corners of the uterus to the pubic area will kink and go into a spasm.
- In the later months, lower groin pressure may develop. Exercising daily can help to alleviate this condition.

Headaches

Useful Exercises

- Neck Smiles in a cross-legged or Zen sitting position (p. 72)
- Self-massage of neck and face (p. 188)
- Partner massage (p. 180)
- Alternate Nostril Breathing (p. 21)
- Complete Relaxation for 10-20 minutes (p. 158)
- Baby Visualization (p. 165)

Cautions and Comments

- Drink strong peppermint, rosemary, catnip, or sage tea and lie down for twenty minutes for complete relaxation.
- Avoid foods with MSG (monosodium glutamate) and nitrates (in luncheon meat). Both of these substances can cause headaches in sensitive people.
- Avoid alcoholic beverages, including wine and champagne.
- For sinus headaches, cut down on dairy products in your diet. Increase your intake of citrus fruits and fresh leafy vegetables.
- Consult your doctor or midwife immediately for severe or long-lasting headaches.
- Do not sleep with your head under the covers, for this creates a shortage of oxygen and then a headache.
- Minimize coffee consumption; it often causes headaches in pregnant women.
- Dairy products can cause extra mucous, sinus problems, and often headaches.

Tips and Other Information

- Walk one mile a day while practicing deep breathing.
- Make "Rock the Baby" breath part of your daily routine.
- Press hot, wet towels on your head and face under a hot shower.
- Lightly massage sinus areas on forehead and cheeks to stimulate drainage of sinuses.

Heartburn

Useful Exercises

- Salute to the Child (p. 94)
- Spinal Twist (p. 76)
- "Rock the Baby" breath (p. 19)
- Baby Breath (p. 23)

Cautions and Comments

- Eat 4-6 small meals a day.
- Drink one tablespoon of cream, milk, or buttermilk before eating to coat and soothe stomach.
- Do not take baking soda or Alka Seltzer. Both have a very high salt content, which may cause water retention and swelling.
- Use alcohol and coffee in moderation, for both have been found to contribute to heartburn in pregnant women.
- *Do not eat highly spiced or greasy foods.*

Tips and Other Information

- The burning sensation results from the re-entrance of stomach fluids into the esophagus (food tube) because of the size of the uterus.
- Gelusil, Milk of Magnesia tablets, or Maalox are often recommended, but *check with your doctor or midwife before taking an antacid.*
- Keep moving if heartburn strikes and do some "Rock the Baby" breathing (p. 19).
- Have patience! It ends with the birth of the baby.

Hemorrhoids

Useful Exercises

- Anal Lock, in Basic Nine (p. 88)
- Pelvic Floor Exercises (p. 89)
- Cross-legged Sitting Position and Rocking (p. 121)
- Salute to the Child (p. 94)

Cautions and Comments

- Increase roughage in your diet to soften stools and make elimination easier. Foods that increase roughage are: raw vegetables, fruits, dried fruits, whole bran flakes, whole grain breads.
- Drink 6-8 glasses of liquid a day (water, juices, herbal teas and milk).
- Hard stools may be quite painful and cause bleeding.
- Do not stay on the toilet bowl for too long. Eliminate and then leave. Make your living room your reading room, not the bathroom.

Tips and Other Information

- Practice the Anal Lock in the shower (p. 88). Fold a washcloth until it is 4″ x 1″. Wet the cloth and wring it out. Place the washcloth on the hemorrhoidal area and practice the Anal Lock. You should be able to hold the washcloth there. Relax the muscles and let the washcloth drop. Repeat 5-10 times.
- Keep your feet and legs elevated on a high footstool while eliminating. This helps to move the bowels by releasing the anal muscles.
- Use cold witch hazel compresses while you elevate your hips on some pillows. With your compress in place, practice the Anal Lock. The witch hazel will help shrink the hemorrhoids and the semi-inverted position will help get the excess blood circulating more effectively.
- Walking one mile a day helps digestion and elimination.

- Keep the bowel area clean by washing completely with warm water after each bowel movement. Then apply oil or A&D ointment.
- Soak in a warm, cold or tepid bath. Afterwards, apply an anesthetic gel such as Anusol to shrink hemorrhoids. *Always check with your caregiver before using any medications during pregnancy.*

Insomnia

Useful Exercises

- Salute to the Child: 2-5 repetitions (p. 94)
- A warm bath before bedtime can help you feel drowsy. Turn the lights down low or take a bath by candlelight.

Cautions and Comments

- Drink hot milk with honey or molasses half an hour before going to bed.
- Herb teas such as camomile, marjoram, and lemon balm are known for their sleep-inducing qualities. Try a hot cup of tea with honey or lemon before bed or in the middle of the night.
- A Vitamin B deficiency in your diet can often cause insomnia. Increase your intake of foods rich in Vitamin B. Keeping a food diary can help diagnose this situation.
- *Do not take any sleeping pills when you are pregnant.*
- Do not force yourself to sleep if you are not really tired. Read or do quiet chores until you feel sleepy.

Tips and Other Information

- Insomnia is very common during the last weeks of pregnancy, when finding a comfortable sleeping position is difficult.
- This is a natural way to prepare for the 3:00 A.M. feeding!
- Arranging pillows behind or under your tummy to relieve breathlessness can be very helpful.

Leg Cramps

Useful Exercises

- Salute to the Child #4, #8, and #10 (p. 94)
- All squatting postures
- Foot Circles (p. 131)
- Foot Rolls (p. 131)

Cautions and Comments

- Increase calcium and potassium intake by including a banana, half a grapefruit, or an orange as a snack. Sesame seeds are high in calcium; sprinkle them on your salad.
- Increase your calcium intake by including some of the following foods in your diet: cottage cheese, ice cream, yogurt, salmon, sardines, soybeans, almonds, sesame seeds.
- Do not stand in one place for too long. Shift your weight from one leg to the other.
- Do not point your toes; point your heel instead.

Tips and Other Information

- Leg cramps are caused by the slowing of your blood circulation.
- Walking one mile a day will help.
- Elevate the legs higher than the heart to prevent cramps.
- When you have a cramp, a hot water bottle or heating pad may help.
- Putting pressure on the cramping area with your hands may bring relief.

Mood Changes

Useful Exercises

- Practicing the PPF program and breathing techniques for 20-30 minutes a day can minimize this problem.
- "Rock the Baby" breath—make it smooth and quiet (p. 19)
- Alternate Nostril Breathing (p. 21)
- Baby Breath (p. 23)
- Baby Visualization (for twenty minutes a day)

Cautions and Comments

- Using your food diary, check to see if you are eating enough foods containing B Vitamins. A shortage of these vitamins can cause depression.
- Check your diet to see that it contains enough iron. Inadequate iron intake causes anemia, which can make you feel tired, irritable and unhappy.

Tips and Other Information

- Mood swings are thought to be caused by hormonal changes. They are quite common in pregnancy. Do not be alarmed.

Nausea

Useful Exercises

- Chest Expansion, standing (p. 90)
- Baby Breath (p. 23)

Cautions and Comments

- Ten mg. per day of Vitamin B6 can help prevent nausea. Once nausea has started, use 25 mg. with each meal. Bananas are a good source of Vitamin B6.
- Eat 4-6 small meals a day. Snack often.
- Red Raspberry leaf, basil, ginger, or peppermint tea all help to eliminate nausea. Use one teaspoon of tea for one cup of hot water, or use tea bags.
- Keep some whole wheat crackers or dry whole wheat toast near your bed. Before getting up, eat the crackers and do a fifteen-minute Complete Relaxation (p. 0). Then get up slowly.
- Cold drinks, such as ginger ale, may help. Do not drink diet cola, since this is high in caffeine and salt.
- Avoid coffee and refined greasy or spicy foods.
- Avoid highly acidic foods (like orange juice in the morning).
- Do not go without eating or drinking because of nausea.
- If the problem persists, speak to your doctor or midwife about it.

Tips and Other Information

- Nausea usually lasts only during the first trimester of pregnancy.
- Nausea is caused by a high estrogen level in the body and the rapid growth of the uterus.
- Have patience. Eventually it will go away.

Nosebleeds and Nasal Congestion

Useful Exercises

- Apply pressure on either side of your nose and between your eyebrows with your fingers. Steadily apply firm pressure, massaging for at least one minute. Shortly thereafter, you should begin to feel drainage.

Cautions and Comments

- Use nose drops or nasal sprays sparingly. Instead, use an empty nasal spray container filled with warm water to spray your nose. This will help to moisten your nose and shrink your membranes.
- If your house tends to be dry, use a humidifier.
- Increase your intake of Vitamin C rich foods such as peppers, cabbage, oranges, lemons, grapefruits, strawberries, and broccoli.
- Dairy products tend to be mucous-producing. Supplement your diet with Dolomite, calcium and magnesium, or bone meal while decreasing dairy product consumption.

Tips and Other Information

- Increased blood volume often causes some capillaries to rupture and causes a nosebleed.
- Lack of Vitamin C may be a contributing factor.
- Nasal jelly in the tip of each nostril may help.
- Stuffiness will disappear with the birth of the baby.
- During pregnancy, inner nasal passages normally swell.

Sciatica

Useful Exercises

- Try all exercises. *Be careful*. If any exercise hurts, do not practice it.

Cautions and Comments

- The sciatic nerve is the largest nerve in the body arising from the sacral plexus, leaving the pelvis through the greater sciatic foramen, running through the hip joint and down the back of the thigh.
- Sciatic nerve irritation is common during pregnancy.

Tips and Other Information

- If you are having problems with sciatica, have your caregiver direct you to either a registered physical therapist or a chiropractor who have been specially trained to deal with pregnancy problems. Usually, working with either a chiropractor or RPT will improve the condition. The birth of your baby usually eliminates this condition entirely.

Skin Problems

Useful Exercises

- The Bridge (p. 81)
- Keep skin clean by washing often with a mild soap

Cautions and Comments

- Taking 5 mg. of Folic Acid (a B Vitamin) before each meal may help pregnancy mask to disappear. (Pregnancy masks are dark blotches on the skin of the face.)
- Do not use make-up is skin is broken out. Use water-based make-up, if you need to wear any at all.

Tips and Other Information

- Skin changes experienced during pregnancy will disappear after the baby is born.
- Common skin problems are pimples, acne, red marks, and mask of pregnancy.

Stitch or Soreness in Rib Area

Useful Exercises

- Chest Expansion (p. 90)
- Salute to the Child #2 and #11 (p. 94)
- Alternate Leg Stretch to the Side (p. 119)

Cautions and Comments

- Avoid Half Sit-Up (in Basic Nine, p. 86) and other postures which increase pressure on this area.

Tips and Other Information

- This often disappears in the last six weeks of pregnancy, once the baby drops into position to be born.
- You should change positions often.

Stretch Marks

Useful Exercises

- Salute to the Child (p. 94) and the Basic Nine (p. 71) help to keep skin in good tone.

Cautions and Comments

- Do not get depressed and think that your tummy has turned into a road map!
- Keep your protein intake high and make sure you are eating foods from the four basic food groups daily.

Tips and Other Information

- Most pregnant women experience stretch marks, so you are in good company.
- Use naturally-cold, pressed vegetable oils such as sesame to keep your skin supple. Massage (with oil) your abdomen, hips, and any other area that seems to be stretching.
- Light-haired people with very sensitive skin should oil and massage their skin daily.
- Red marks turn pale silver or white after the baby is born. They never disappear completely, but they do become much less noticeable.

Sweating

Useful Exercises

- "Rock the Baby" breath (p. 19), focusing on the coolness of the air coming into your body and the warmth of the air leaving it
- Complete Relaxation (p. 158). When you relax completely, your body tends to feel cooler.

Cautions and Comments

- Your body is making sure that its temperature is perfect for your baby's development. Dress accordingly.
- Do not use a hot tub during pregnancy. This increase in body temperature can often cause your baby to go into fetal distress.

Tips and Other Information

- •Wear loose, comfortable clothing (as if you have a choice!) throughout your pregnancy.
- •Dress lightly. Even though it is cold outside, you may feel warm.
- •Think about how much money you're saving on heating bills!

Swelling (Edema) of Hands and Feet

Useful Exercises

- •Easy sitting posture (p. 121)
- •Zen sitting position (p. 102)
- •Sitting on a Seiza bench (p. 126)
- •Ankle Rotation, for swollen ankles (p. 131)
- •Deep breathing with your legs at a 45° angle against the wall for 3-5 minutes

Cautions and Comments

- •Do not eat highly salted foods such as potato chips, crackers, pretzels, salted peanuts, etc.
- •Do *not* eliminate *all* salt from your diet. Keep salt consumption at a moderate level by preparing your own foods rather than using premixed, processed, or canned foods.
- •Eat a well-balanced, high-protein diet.
- •Tell your doctor about this condition as soon as you notice it. It can be the first stage of toxemia, which is a very serious disease of pregnancy.
- •Follow your doctor's or midwife's directions precisely.
- •Do not take diuretics (water pills) when you are pregnant.
- •Do not sit with a weight, such as another child, on your legs. This impedes your circulation.

Tips and Other Information

- •A rise in estrogen in the body causes swelling in pregnancy. Some swelling is to be expected and is acceptable.
- •Hands, legs, and feet may get puffy and swollen. Remove your rings when you notice this condition. Do not wait, or the rings may have to be cut off.
- •Wear loose, comfortable clothing.
- •Walking one mile a day helps to keep this condition under control.
- •Be sure to wear properly-fitting shoes, which may be larger than your normal size. Once the baby arrives, your feet will return to normal.

Urination (Frequent)

Useful Exercises

- Anal Lock (p. 88)
- Pelvic Floor Exercise (p. 89)

Cautions and Comments

- Do not cut down on your fluid intake. Drink 6-8 glasses of fluid a day.

Tips and Other Information

- Nightly trips to the bathroom prepare you for upcoming nightly trips to the baby's room.
- This is a natural by-product of the early and late months of pregnancy.
- Hang your favorite picture or photo in the bathroom so you have something pleasant to look at.

Varicose Veins

Useful Exercises

- Salute to the Child, #8 (p. 94)
- Basic Nine Leg Lifts on the side (p. 84)
- Leg Cradles (p. 74)
- Sitting on a Seiza bench (p. 126)
- For Vaginal Varicosities: Assume a position on your back as shown in Figure 4.1. Hold onto a chair and place your feet on the seat of the chair. Lift your bottom up into the air and hold it there for fifteen seconds to one minute, breathing normally. Immediately lower your legs to the side of the chair and take 1-2 "Rock the Baby" (p. 19) breaths (see Figure 4.2). Get up when you are ready.
- Complete Relaxation, with legs elevated on two pillows, or on the seat part of a chair, or on a 45° angle against the wall

Cautions and Comments

- Do not wear restrictive socks (knee socks), garters, or belts.
- Do not wear high-heeled shoes.
- Do not stand for long periods of time.
- Do not sit in cross-legged positions.

Tips and Other Information

- Varicose veins are enlarged veins close to the surface of the skin. They usually disappear after the birth of the baby.
- Walking one mile a day is very helpful.
- Wear support hose if your doctor or midwife recommends them. Keep them near your bed and put them on before you get out of bed in the morning.
- As often as you can, sit with your feet up higher than your heart.
- Change positions frequently.
- The recommended position for dealing with vaginal varicosities will drain your vaginal area of accumulated blood and may temporarily relieve the condition.

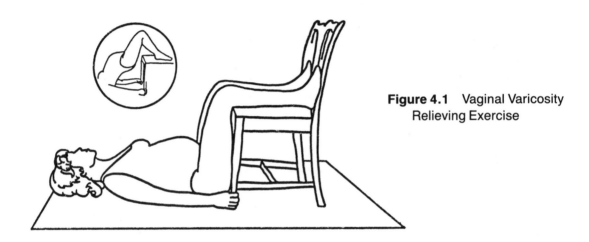

Figure 4.1   Vaginal Varicosity Relieving Exercise

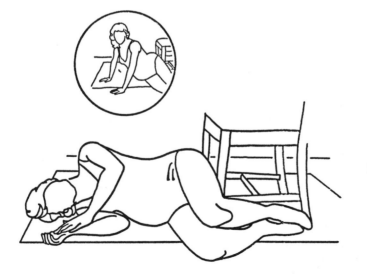

Figure 4.2   After the Exercise

CHAPTER FIVE:

The Many Moods of Pregnancy

"I just don't feel like myself.....I'm so moody. One moment I'm crying, often for no apparent reason, and the next minute I'm laughing. Then there are days when I am even-tempered and calm. These mood swings are so unpredictable, I feel like I'm on an emotional roller coaster. Little things bother me that I wouldn't have even thought about before my pregnancy. The people and the daily events in my life even seem to have changed. I can empathize with people and events much more than I used to. This depth of feeling is a new experience for me."

This quote was taken from a letter I received from a pregnant friend who thought I might be able to reassure her that all these changes and new revelations were normal outcroppings of the pregnancy experience. I told her that the emotional reactions experienced during the waiting months are as varied as the women. They reflect the woman's physical and mental state at the time. The reactions continually change as the pregnancy progresses. However, I did reassure my friend that she was still "normal."

Some of my students do not report any noticeable changes in their emotional state, while others experience new depths and intensities of emotion. Many women report a strong "nesting instinct," which imparts a feeling of calm and protection. Although there is no definite pattern, it is important to be aware of the possibility of heightened emotions during your pregnancy. If you think about all the physical and hormonal changes that naturally occur within your body as the baby develops, it becomes apparent that they will have some effect on your mental attitudes and emotions. Students have often been awed by the sheer power of their emotions. The emotional control you had prior to your pregnancy may disappear. This can be very scary, since we rely heavily on past conditioning to solve today's problems or handle complex situations.

THE CONNECTION BETWEEN MOOD AND BODY

Bodily changes during pregnancy are often accompanied by changes in emotions. Your own personal reaction to your body's growth, shape, and proportions may be a source of pride one day and upset the next. It is believed that these changes are related to the increase in the progesterone level in the pregnant body. Many women are moody or irritable just before the onset of their monthly period, when this same hormone is at a very high level. Thus, the hormone can affect you in the same way during pregnancy.

ANCIENT EXPLANATIONS

In the past, studies were done to try to understand human development. Current psychological studies examine the effect of daily stressors or changes on the body and mind. However, since the conclusions of these current studies are often in conflict with one another, let's turn instead to the findings of the ancient yogis of India. They were essentially looking for answers to the same questions that puzzle us today. The model that they created thousands of years ago may be of some help to your understanding of your own emotional state during pregnancy.

From a yogic point of view, everything within the universe contains life force, or inner energy. When the female body is in the process of nurturing a new human being, this life force increases. The increase in this level of inner energy often causes an increase in emotional reactions. Perhaps inner energy is the basic ingredient from which we create emotions. According to the writings of the ancient yogis, your life force is the one aspect of you which will never die. During pregnancy, you are really in a state of heightened vitality and life. You may be more sensitive to people, react more strongly to events, taste food with more clarity, and even sense things before they happen. You are more alive!

As you read this, however, you may be thinking, "If I am so much more alive, how come I am always so tired?" That is a very valid question. There is a big difference between inner energy and the energy that is used for daily physical activities. Ancient yogic writings contain a description of another, subtle body within our physical body. There is no counterpart to this idea in modern Western medicine. The subtle body contains the channels through which our life force flows. The yogis described seven energy centers or "chakras," from the bottom of your spine to the top of your head, each of which has a special relationship with this inner realm. The chakras can be thought of as the connectors between our inner nature and our physical body. During pregnancy, when there is an increased output of inner energy, you may become more aware of the manifestations of the different chakras.

The *first chakra* is thought to be located in the perineum and is called the root chakra. It is concerned with the survival of the human body. The *second chakra*, located in the spine in the small of the back, is usually associated with sexual function. The *third chakra*, located in the spine just above the navel, is associated with the human drives for achieving power, fame, glory, and prestige. The *fourth chakra*, located in the spine behind the heart, is associated with love and compassion toward our fellow human beings. The *fifth chakra*, located in the spine at the base of the neck, is associated with oral and written communication. The *sixth chakra*, located between the eyebrows, is concerned with seeing people as they really are, rather than how they appear to be. The *seventh chakra*, located at the top of the head, is the connecting point between energy within the body and energy outside the body (see Figure 5.1).

When inner energy flows through you, your perceptions and experiences of life change. This is particularly evident during pregnancy. For example, many expectant mothers report feeling "protected" by a higher power or force. This is a very definite manifestation of the seventh chakra, which is associated with a sense of spiritual awakening or awareness. Other women have been frightened by a feeling of pressure in the head. This is a manifestation of the sixth and seventh chakras. A feeling of pressure in the chest, as well as an increase in feelings of compassion, is related to the fourth chakra. Any gut feelings in your stomach may be related to the lower chakras. You may sometimes experience emotions so deep, you can almost taste them. These are associated with the fifth chakra. Some mothers have accurate visions of what their babies will look like, or be like. This is a manifestation of the sixth chakra.

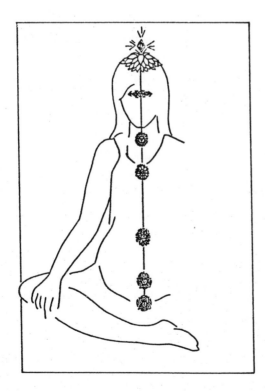

Figure 5.1   The Seven "Chakras"
or Energy Centers,
With Their Ancient Symbols

A PLAN FOR COPING

All these characteristics of the chakras are simply indications of your higher potential and nature, which become quite evident for some women during pregnancy. Because the experiences are so vivid, you may begin to question your own sanity and, therefore, react in a negative way. Normally, there are two methods for dealing with heightened and turbulent emotions: you can *retreat from* the emotions, or *respond to* the emotions. However, during pregnancy the second method is usually the one chosen. Since most of your conditioning up until now has probably been along the lines of retreating from the emotion, at first you may have some difficulty adjusting to this new response. However, there are some helpful hints which can put this theory to practical use. It's easy to say, "Oh, that's my fourth chakra acting up" when you find yourself in tears over a TV program. But when you are in a rage while your in-laws are visiting, it's a different story. The following plan of action for the many moods of pregnancy can be most useful to you:

1. Discuss your feelings openly with your mate. Talk about the heightened emotions, your helplessness, and your need for some emotional support. Keep the lines of communication open throughout the pregnancy.

2. Keep a journal of your feelings. Use a small notebook to write down how you feel, why you think you feel that way, etc. Be honest about your feelings, writing down the negative ones as well. Try the "Turn the Leaf Over" (pp. 62-63) exercise in the journal as well as in your thinking processes. Pretend that you are a pregnant character in a play—your life—and look for the character's motivations. What daily lessons is she learning in her life?

3. Go with your emotions. Suppressing them will not be useful; you may not always be able to do it, anyway, and you may begin to feel guilty. Let the emotions ride over and through you. Really *feel* love, hate, anger, fear, and depression. Imagine that there is a door at the top of your head, and let the emotion ride all the way up the spine (that is the shortest route in the later months) and out the door. Take two or three "Rock the Baby" breaths (p. 19) when the power of the emotion leaves.

4. Even if you feel lazy, practice your PPF exercises as often as you can. These exercises will stimulate and activate your inner energy to flow smoothly and freely along your inner passageways. They will help you to become calm, flexible, and strong while physically energizing you.

5. During the last weeks of your pregnancy, you may notice an increase in anxieties as you fantasize about the forthcoming birth. You may wonder if your child will be born vaginally or if it will be a Cesarean section (C/Sec) birth. You may find yourself particularly worried about the baby's health or whether you will be able

to endure the labor process. Sometimes it seems as though this pregnancy will go on forever, especially if your baby is overdue. Because you never really know when labor will begin, just going to the store and fearing that your water will break can be an anxiety-ridden experience. Your natural "nesting instinct" causes you to plan and worry about the future. Thoughts such as "Will I be a good parent?" or "Will I be able to support this child?" may run through your head. But *you cannot know what the future will hold until you are living in it*. Wasteless energy is expended worrying about what might or might not happen. When your brain is in turmoil, the wisest course of action to choose is to stop everything, sit down in a comfortable chair, and *relax*.

6.   Practice calming breaths, such as Alternate Nostril Breath (p. 21) and Smooth Breath (pp. 25-26). If you practice breathing for 2-3 minutes, it can change your whole perspective.

7.   Practice Relaxation and Visualization for 15-20 minutes twice a day on a regular basis to have a positive outlet for your fantasies (see Chapter 8).

8.   Find out if any PPF classes are being offered in your community. By enrolling in these or other early and mid-pregnancy programs, you will be able to share your experiences with other people. You will make many friends who will lend a sympathetic ear. The class will probably become a support group for you.

9.   Share your emotions mentally with your baby. Since he or she bears the brunt of these emotions while living inside your agitated or depressed body, you may as well include him in a discussion of it. Be honest with the baby. Anger is just as much a part of mothering as love. Children seem to instinctively understand this. An incident comes to mind that will illustrate my point. For some reason which I cannot recall, I had yelled at my older son, Mathew, who was about five years old at the time. He already knew how to write, so he went to his room, made the following note, and gave it to me: "I still love you even when your (sic) mad." I still have that note, for the message is one we all need to remember from time to time.

10.   Accept you heightened sensitivity as Nature's way of preparing you for your forthcoming mothering role. You will need heightened ESP to know how to communicate with a screaming baby who is neither hungry nor sleepy at 3:00 A.M.! Accepting and going with the situation rather than fighting it can be a valuable part of your training for motherhood.

11.   During times of extremely heightened emotions, you may forget to eat, or may eat whatever is handy (i.e., junk food). Emotion quickly burns up the B Vitamins that are in your body. Since the body cannot manufacture B Vitamins and therefore depends on your diet for an adequate supply, you must remain aware of what you are eating. If you get into the habit of snacking on B Vitamin-rich foods such as sunflower, pumpkin, or sesame seeds, you will not experience depression due to

a lack of these vitamins. But although B Vitamins do play a role in emotional stability, only a balanced diet chosen wisely from the four basic food groups will ensure total physical and mental well-being. Remember to eat 5-6 small meals a day to minimize nausea as well as emotional upsets.

One final, and pleasant, note. You'll probably find that people are more friendly and helpful when you are pregnant. Strangers may open doors for you, carry packages, or ask when your baby is due. Enjoy this special treatment, since most of it will shift over to the baby when he arrives. Combine this special treatment with a mental attitude of increased inner vitality, increased health, increased creativity, and new life. Allow yourself to be open to the many new experiences that can be yours during these waiting months. Indeed, you are *most* alive when you are in this state of creation.

CHAPTER SIX
Fear Is a Four-Letter Word

Of all the topics discussed in my classes, none is more common than the fears associated with pregnancy, birth, and motherhood. Where do these fears come from?

Maybe your mother talked to you about her negative birth experience. Maybe your best friend kept questioning her ability to cope. In any event, it really doesn't matter *where* you first acquired these fears. It is, however, most important that you *now* become aware of your fears and do something to overcome them.

"What are your biggest fears during pregnancy?" My students usually respond to this question with silence. Everyone looks around; no one wants to admit her fear. Then some brave soul quietly verbalizes her fear of not having a normal child. Quickly, the group becomes very vocal. One student usually says, "Oh, you have that fear too?" As soon as it becomes obvious that the primary fears during pregnancy are fairly universal, everyone sighs with relief. Then the discussion can really progress.

"What should you do with your fears?" is usually the next question raised. Throughout the ensuing discussion, it becomes apparent that sharing your fears with others in the same situation helps to make those fears diminish or, in some cases, disappear.

One conclusion that is often reached during these talks relates to facing your fears. We have found that *not* facing your fears headlong can produce pain and suffering, while doing the opposite—leveling with yourself and the group—helps to eradicate the fear. The group is always happy to find out that 95% of all babies born in this country at the present time are perfectly normal. So the odds are certainly in your favor!

This leads to a second, very important, point: most fear thrives in ignorance. Many fears are based on your imaginary understanding of a situation rather than a factual one. If, for example, a student is afraid of being in the hospital, I usually suggest a tour of the local hospital to see all the areas which she may be using for labor, birth, and confinement. If the hospital is still not agreeable to her, then she and her husband might explore the idea of a home birth. The options are there, but you must first know what you are fighting.

Another extremely important point that usually emerges from these group discussions is that help is available in most instances when you really need it. I continually emphasize in my classes that the pregnant woman will receive help. When my students accept the fact that their cries for help will be heard and answered, many of their fears disappear.

Worrying, rather than dealing with fear, makes the emotion grow totally out of proportion. Many women spend their whole pregnancy worrying about what will go wrong. What a waste of energy! Instead, use these nine months to develop physically, mentally, and emotionally for the child to come.

The PPF program can help you to be totally aware of your feelings and experiences during the waiting time. Once your fears are recognized, you should talk about them. "Great," you may say, "but I don't happen to have a class or group to talk to." Remember that there are always people to talk to. Perhaps you can talk with your husband, doctor, midwife, or a friend.

The positive experience of sharing time and feelings with other pregnant women seems to help allay fears. One of the most beneficial parts of PPF is the socializing that goes on between women in the same situation. Find out if there is a group like this in your area. Perhaps you could start your own informal group.

Learning to recognize, admit, and face your feelings will make your pregnancy a more positive experience. There is a very simple PPF mental exercise that is most beneficial for dealing with your fears once you have pinpointed them. This mental exercise is called "Turn Over the Leaf."

Imagine that each one of your fears is a leaf with two very different sides (see Figure 6.1):

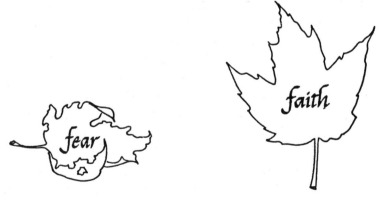

Figure 6.1   The Leaf

Side 1: FEAR		Side 2: FAITH
This side reads: "I will never be able to make it through labor and delivery."	TURN IT OVER	The other side reads: "I will have the inner strength and help I need to have a good birth experience."
Or: "I will not be able to take care of the baby once it arrives."	TURN IT OVER	"I am going to educate myself by reading books and talking to other new mothers. I may not have all the answers, but I will do the best I can."
Or: "I will not be able to cope with all the new responsibilities."	TURN IT OVER	"I have faith in myself and I know I can do a good job. I will get help when I need it."

Whenever your head is filled with fears about the baby or your new motherhood role, you have to remember to turn over the leaf. For a concrete reminder of this exercise, go out into the woods and select a healthy, strong-looking leaf. Bring the leaf home with you and simply take two sheets of wax paper, put the leaf between them, and iron the wax paper together. Be sure the iron is on a very low setting. Then hang the leaf in a place that you pass frequently. The leaf will be a tangible reminder to keep the faith!

With some practice, you can learn to keep away from the power of negative thinking and concentrate instead on the positive. The most rewarding benefit of this mental exercise is a better knowledge and understanding of the workings of your brain.

Your mental attitude contributes to your child's inner environment. The baby shares your body, and thus experiences many of your feelings. A positive attitude will contribute to both your and the baby's enjoyment of this new adventure.

CHAPTER SEVEN
Exercises for All the Pregnant Months

PRACTICE GUIDELINES

During pregnancy your body is constantly changing and growing on the *inside* as well as on the outside. Therefore, the exercises you do have to change and adapt to your growing shape and weight. Many of the exercises you may have done before the advent of the baby can be continued all during the pregnant months, with the agreement of your doctor or midwife. But when and if these forms of exercise become uncomfortable or straining to you, they should be minimized or eliminated completely. A brisk, daily, one-mile walk can be easily substituted for the more strenuous exercises.

The idea that you should do nothing physical for nine months because you are in a "delicate condition" is no longer fashionable or acceptable. In fact, it is becoming more evident that a total exercise and relaxation program throughout the full nine months of pregnancy often facilitates the birth experience. Quite simply, you will feel better after you have begun to practice the PPF program.

For your convenience, a set of "Basic Nine" exercises has been developed: these postures should be the backbone of your exercise program. All nine exercises can and should be used throughout the pregnancy. Also included here is a creative series of twelve interwoven positions called "Salute to the Child." It is advisable to use "Rock the Baby" breath (p. 19) or Baby Breath (p. 23) during your practice sessions. What follows are some basic instructions for doing all the exercises.

1. Take one or two "Rock the Baby" or Baby Breaths.

2. Slowly assume the chosen position. Relax those muscles you are not directly stretching.

3. Hold and stretch, trying to remain still for as long as possible.

4. Slowly return to your starting position.

5. Take one or two more "Rock the Baby" or Baby Breaths.

6. Follow with another exercise or a Relaxation position and more breathing.

7. *Keep your mental awareness at all times on the physical feelings of your movements, on your breathing, or on your baby.*

If you disregard these directions and race through the PPF exercises, thinking about what you will make for dinner or what you are going to do next week, all of your efforts will be wasted and may, in fact, do you some harm. To make these postures work for you, they must be done *slowly*, with total concentration. The unification of your mind, body, and breath will ensure success with the program and a more positive, rewarding pregnancy.

Do's and Don'ts of Prenatal Fitness

Do check with your doctor or midwife before beginning any exercise program.

Do try to be consistent in the amount of time you practice—20-30 minutes a day is fine.

Do wear loose, comfortable clothing—leotards are not necessary and can cause a urinary tract infection.

Do practice floor exercises on a comfortable foam mat or indoor/outdoor carpet.

Do try to practice sitting cross-legged or squatting daily. If you have varicose veins, these positions should *not* be practiced.

Do try to move gracefully and easily from one exercise to another.

Do breathe deeply before and after each exercise. Use "Rock the Baby" breath (p. 19).

Do keep your mind on what you are feeling as you stretch and relax. Tune into your body and your baby.

Do stretch as far as you can comfortably and then relax into the posture. Make sure all muscle groups not being used are relaxed.

Do end your practice session with several abdominal breaths and a complete relaxation.

Do practice relaxation/visualization daily to communicate with your child.

Do have a positive attitude about yourself and your baby.

Do enjoy the miracle of pregnancy and birth!!

Don't get into pain while practicing. Go to the *edge* of pain, not *into* it.

Don't rush through an exercise session. Take your time and tune in.

Don't practice the following exercises during pregnancy:

- Double leg lifts—strain lower back and abdominal muscles
- Regular sit-ups—strain lower back; can contribute to separated recti muscles
- Inverted postures such as shoulder-stand and headstand—cause excess blood to rush to head, causing headaches
- Violent stomach contractions such as yoga abdominal lifts—cut off oxygen supply to baby and body
- Exercises which begin with pregnant woman lying flat on stomach

Don't let your head hang forward when doing forward bending exercises. Instead, keep your chin up. Regular forward bends sometimes cause fainting from the excessive blood rush to the head.

Don't practice in a poorly-ventilated room. Make sure there is plenty of air circulation.

Don't wear shoes when practicing stretching exercises. Feel the mat or ground with your toes.

Don't lie on your back for extended periods of time after the fifth month of pregnancy. When back-lying, bend your knees, place your feet on the floor hip distance apart to take pressure off the lower back (lumbar spine). Flat back-lying cuts off the blood return to the torso from the legs by allowing the heavy uterus to lie on the vena cava. Flat back-lying will also cause a drop in oxygen supply to the baby.

Don't practice two back-lying exercises in a row. Instead, practice one back-lying, follow with a side-lying pose, and then go back to back-lying.

Don't practice exercises which include hopping, bouncing, or jumping. These movements may cause pain or strain in the lower back, hip and pelvic joints, in addition to straining the pelvic floor (Kegel) muscles.

Don't exercise when you are ill. At those times, practice only breathing, centering, talking to the baby and relaxation.

Don't overheat the body and thus raise the normal body temperature. This will often cause the baby to go into fetal distress. *Avoid saunas and hot tubs.*

Don't hold your breath during exercise routines. This cuts off oxygen to both baby and Mom's body.

Don't point toes excessively during pregnancy. This tends to cause calf cramps. Instead, flex the foot pointing your toes toward the knee or leading with the heel.

Don't practice exercises right after eating. Wait at least 1-2 hours.

Don't fast during pregnancy. This loss of calories and nourishment is harmful to both mother and baby.

Don't take chances during pregnancy. If you are in doubt, consult your doctor or midwife for correct advice.

Don't practice prenatal exercises without total medical consent if you have any one of the following conditions: high blood pressure, diabetes, preeclampsia, toxemia, prior history of miscarriage or premature labor, placenta privia, any vaginal bleeding, persistent dizziness, headache, breathlessness, or nausea.

Warning Signs During Pregnancy

If you experience any of the following symptoms, immediately discontinue the PPF program and consult your doctor or midwife:

- •extreme pain
- •vaginal bleeding
- •dizziness
- •faintness
- •shortness of breath
- •palpitations
- •back and pubic pain
- •difficulty walking

Your symptoms may be non-conclusive, but you are much better off getting a professional opinion.

Preterm Labor

You should be forewarned about preterm labor just in case it happens to you. A normal pregnancy takes forty weeks to complete. Preterm labor occurs after the twentieth week but before the thirty-seventh week. It is a condition in which uterine contractions (tightening of the womb) cause the cervix (mouth of the womb) to thin out and open earlier than usual. It could result in the birth of a preterm baby.

The cause of preterm labor is unknown, but you can prevent a preterm birth by being aware of the warning symptoms. These are uterine contractions that occur ten minutes apart or closer with or without the following:

- •menstrual-like cramps in the lower abdomen and above the pubic bone, which may be erratic or constant
- •a low, dull backache below the waistline that may be erratic or constant
- •pelvic pressure that feels like your baby is pushing down—it may be erratic
- •abdominal cramping with or without diarrhea
- •an increase or change in vaginal discharge that results in a mucousy, watery, or light bloody discharge

It is quite normal to have some uterine contractions throughout the day. These usually occur when you are changing positions. It is *not* normal, however, to have frequent uterine contractions that occur every ten minutes for 1-2 hours. Such uterine contractions may cause your cervix to open too early.

If you think you are experiencing preterm labor, lie down and *tilt toward* your left side, placing a pillow at your back for support. Place your fingers on your uterus and time your contractions with a clock that has a second hand. Time the contractions from the beginning of one contraction to the beginning of the next. Sometimes, lying down for an hour may make the symptoms go away. If you discover a regular pattern of contractions after one hour, call your doctor or midwife immediately. Medications are now available for the treatment of preterm labor, but early identification is the key.

Good Posture vs. Bad Posture

Since pregnancy may be a new experience for you, you have to take some comfort measures. You should try to tune into your body more and become aware of your posture. Good posture is essential for the pregnant woman's health and well-being.

Study Figure 7.1 very carefully and you will see the "pregnancy slouch." This is characterized by:

- an over-exaggerated curve of the back to compensate for the extra weight in front
- a distortion of the whole spine
- flabby thighs, buttocks and abdomen

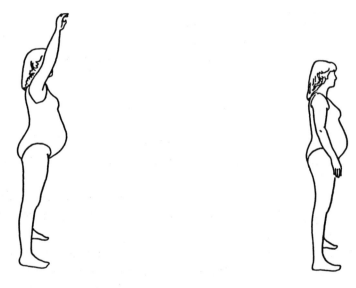

Figure 7.1   BAD Pregnancy Posture   **Figure 7.2**   GOOD Pregnancy Posture

The direct result of "pregnancy slouch" is *backache*, *pain* and *stiffness*. But there is no reason to suffer like that during your pregnancy. Study Figure 7.2 to see how you *should* be standing. Look at yourself in front of a mirror so you can correct your own posture, or get your mate or a friend to help you.

Good posture is characterized by:

- A well-balanced head that doesn't compress your neck. The back of the neck should lengthen upward. Pretend that there is a string pulling your head toward the ceiling.
- Your shoulders are relaxed, thereby draining tension from the shoulders, neck, and upper back.
- Your spine is lengthened, providing plenty of space for the growing baby.
- Your abdominal muscles do not sag but act as a strong corset to support the growing weight of your baby inside.
- Your pelvis is correctly placed so that both the abdomen and the buttocks can help support the lower body effectively. You will also be preventing lower back strain.

Lifting and Bending During Pregnancy

Your daily movements have to be changed during pregnancy because of your added weight and the extra progesterone in your body that makes your ligaments, muscles, and joints looser. When you practice the PPF program, you will automatically lengthen your spine. There are, however, some precautions that you should take:

- Always bend your knees, *not your back*.
- Bend down into a squat whenever you need to reach down.
- Brace your pelvic floor muscles and abdominal muscles before lifting any heavy objects, including children.

Tips For Pregnancy Comfort

Harmony and comfort during pregnancy depends on your adjusting your movements as the pregnancy progresses. You must constantly adjust to your changing center of gravity.

When doing the dishes, place one foot on a low stool for five minutes and then switch feet on the stool. This maneuver releases tension in your lower back, thereby preventing pregnancy backache (see Figure 7.3).

When sitting, try to put your feet up on a stool or on another chair. This maneuver helps the circulation in your legs, thereby making it easier for your body to get your blood pumped back to the heart against the pull of gravity. Put a pillow underneath your knees or calves for greater comfort (see Figure 7.4).

When getting up from a lying-down position, walk yourself up slowly using your hands. If you get up quickly, you may feel faint (see Figure 7.5).

The Guidelines in this section are meant to guide you through your personal pregnancy experience with greater comfort and ease. You should always keep them in mind, not only as you practice the exercises in this book but also as you go about your daily chores.

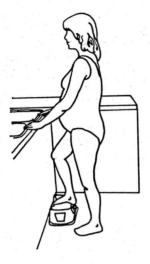

Figure 7.3 Using a Stool to Prevent Pregnancy Backache

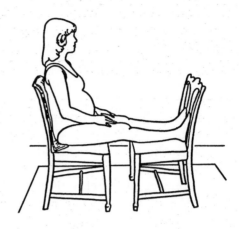

Figure 7.4 Sitting With Your Legs Up

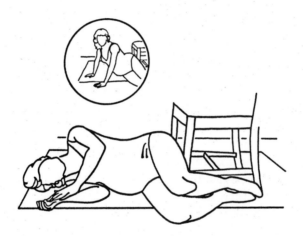

Figure 7.5 Walking Yourself Up Into a Sitting Position

THE "BASIC NINE"

The core of your prenatal exercise routine should be the "Basic Nine." Each of these exercises will benefit your body in a special way, but all will eliminate tension and tiredness from your body and mind. Spend some time early on in your pregnancy learning these simple and enjoyable exercises and you will be rewarded with an almost trouble-free pregnancy. Remember that, as your body grows larger, you will have to make certain changes and allowances while practicing. Do not become discouraged when an exercise that seemed relatively easy in the fifth month becomes more difficult in the eighth or ninth month.

1a. Neck Smiles

Benefits

- Promotes full, pain-free neck motion.
- May relieve pain and tension in the neck.
- Keeps the neck and shoulders loose and limber.
- Encourages the relaxation of facial and jaw muscles—a key to general relaxation.
- Helps to relax the entire body, eliminates insomnia, and prevents headaches.
- Stretches and strengthens all layers of postvertebral muscles in the capital and cervical regions, including: the sternocleidomastoideus, the scalene muscle groups, superficial and deeper erector spinae muscles.

Directions

1. Sit up straight in any comfortable sitting position. Close your eyes, letting your head fall loosely forward with your chin near your chest (see Figure 7.6).

2. Now imagine that your lips are drawing an imaginary smile in the space directly in front of you. Keeping your shoulders still, slowly move your chin until it is directly above your right shoulder. Draw an imaginary straight line from your right shoulder to your left shoulder as you move your head slowly over to the left.

3. Once your chin is above the left shoulder, release the muscles in the back of your neck and allow your chin to come down as close to your body as possible. Draw the imaginary curving bottom of the smile as you move your head from left to right.

4. Repeat the two movements making three smiles, beginning on the right, going across to the left, and returning to the right again. Take about fifteen seconds to draw one smile. Be sure your movements are smooth and fluid.

5. Gracefully move your chin above the left shoulder and make three more neck smiles beginning on the left, going to the right, and then completing the imaginary smile on the left side.

6. Raise your head slowly when your Neck Smiles are completed. Take one "Rock the Baby" breath (p. 19) and relax.

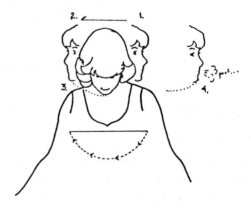

Figure 7.6   Neck Smiles in Various Positions

Cautions and Comments

•Your neck may crack and creak. Don't worry—you are not falling apart! This is perfectly normal and helpful for keeping the neck area—a very popular tension spot—loose and limber.

•Practice this exercise during television commercials or whenever you have a spare moment.

•This exercise is especially helpful for women who work in offices and spend much of their time looking down.

•Neck Smiles are a quick energizer.

1b. Neck Twists

Benefits

•Releases muscular tension in the shoulders and neck.

•Stretches and strengthens the muscles at the sides of the neck, including the sternocleidomastoideus, the scalene muscle group, the longus cervicus and capitus muscles.

•Increases body flexibility and neck range of motion.

Directions

1. Shift your head to the center and up straight, with your eyes closed. Check your facial muscles to make sure they are loose and relaxed. Let your jaw muscles go.

2. Keep your head up straight as you move it as far around to the right side as you can comfortably. Take a breath, purse your lips and blow it out (see Figure 7.6).

3. Now you will find that you can shift your head a bit further to the right. Take another breath, purse your lips and blow it out. Shift again even further to the right.

4. Check to see that your shoulders, jaw and face are loose and relaxed.

5. Take one more breath, stretch a bit further, then release it and come back to center.

6. Repeat these movements on the left side.

7. Return to center and take 1-2 "Rock the Baby" breaths (p. 19). Close your eyes, look inside, center and relax for a few seconds.

Cautions and Comments

•Do not twist so far that you feel pain.

•Do not twist your shoulders, only your head.

•This exercise will make you aware of the power of your breath and how the breath can be used to enhance a movement.

•If you work in an office, practice this exercise 3-4 times a day.

•Remember to keep your neck and shoulders relaxed throughout this exercise.

•Keep your chin tucked to prevent your head from thrusting forward and tightening your shoulder muscles.

2. Leg Cradles

Benefits

- Limbers up the legs, hips, and pelvic area so you can sit more comfortably in a cross-legged position.
- Strengthens your deltoideus muscle group, shoulder rotator cuff group, upper back postvertebral and rhomboideus muscles, oblique abdominal group and quadraceps.
- Loosens tight muscle groups in your thighs and calves.
- Prepares the legs for the pushing stage of labor.
- Strengthens your arms and shoulders while releasing muscular tension.
- Stretches your pectoralis major muscle group, the hip rotators, the gluteal muscle group, the hamstrings, the gastrocnemius-soleus muscle group.

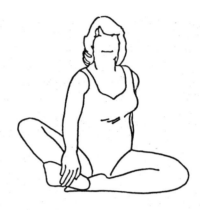

Figure 7.7 Leg Cradles As You Warm Your Leg

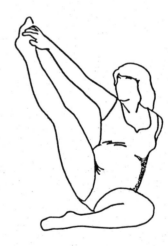

Figure 7.8 Outstretched Leg Movement

Directions

1. Sit in a comfortable cross-legged position with your back unsupported and your head and shoulders straight up.

2. Place your left hand on the mat behind you, fingers facing away from the body. Place your right hand on your right arch (see Figure 7.7).

3. Slowly begin to stretch your leg up into the air and then down again. Repeat 5-10 times to warm up the leg (see Figure 7.8).

4. If you have difficulty straightening out the leg, then hold your leg at the ankle (see Figure 7.9) and repeat the same movements.

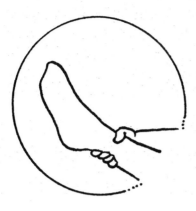

Figure 7.9 Ankle Hold Position

5. Once the leg is warmed up, begin to move it from side to side, stretching it as far as you can to each side, while keeping it fairly straight up in the air. Repeat 5-10 times. Then bend and lower your leg. Take a deep breath and let it go.

6. Place your left hand on your right foot and the right hand on the right knee, lifting the bent leg up (see Figure 7.10).

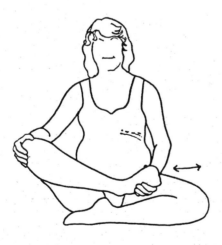

Figure 7.10 Side-to-Side Stretch Position

7. Move it gently from side to side 5-10 times, concentrating on your hip point. Feel warmth in the hip area as you stretch the tensor fasciae (Iliotibial band) and hip external rotators.

8. Place the outer edge of your right foot in the crook of your left elbow and wrap your right arm around the outside of the cradled leg. Clasp your hands in front of your leg if you can (see Figure 7.11). If that is impossible, simply hold your right foot with your left hand and right knee with your right hand.

9. Move the leg from side to side several times in this position, letting the leg do the work.

10. Bring the cradled leg directly in front of you and imagine that the leg is dead weight. Using your left arm, begin to draw imaginary circles in the air with your left elbow. Make 5-10 circles and then reverse for 5-10 circles (see Figure 7.11). Feel a warmth in your left arm and shoulder as you strengthen your upper back post vertebrals, anterior deltoideus, biceps, and pectoralis major. Feel your leg working and stretching as you use your gluteus maximus, hip rotators and hip adductors.

11. Lower your leg to the mat. Take 1-2 "Rock the Baby" breaths (p. 19) and repeat Leg Cradle movements with the left leg. When both legs have been stretched and warmed up, close your eyes, look inside, center and relax for a few seconds.

Cautions and Comments

- This exercise may seem difficult when you first practice it, but in time you will notice your legs becoming more and more limber.
- Keep your knee bent during Direction #5 if it is painful to straighten it out.
- One leg may be much easier to exercise than the other. We tend to have a dominant leg as well as a dominant arm.
- This exercise can be practiced sitting on the floor during television commercials.
- Toward the end of pregnancy, when the abdomen is large, you may not be able to comfortably cradle the leg. Instead, hold the leg with both hands and circle the foot in that position.

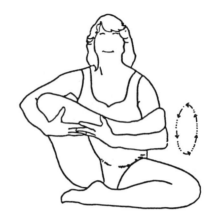

Figure 7.11   Drawing Circles in the Air

3. Pregnancy Spinal Twist

Benefits

- Strengthens the middle, lower back postvertebrals, oblique abdominalis and transverse abdominalis muscles.
- Stretches middle and lower back postvertebrals (erector spinae), oblique abdominalis group, gluteal muscle group.
- Relieves muscular tension and maintains a supple vertebral column.
- Keeps the sides of the growing waistline intact and well-toned.
- Keeps your spine limber and, thereby, has a therapeutic effect on your nervous system.
- Often relieves side stitches in the later months of pregnancy.
- Is an energizing posture for a quick pick-me-up.

Directions

1. Sitting up straight in a cross-legged or open "V" leg position (if you have varicose veins), place your left hand on your right knee.

2. Extend your right arm out straight, with your pinky facing up toward the ceiling. Keeping the arm at shoulder height, gracefully push it as far behind you as you can (see Figure 7.12).

3. Look toward your pinky, keeping your head up straight.

4. Place your right hand down on the mat behind you with your fingers pointing away from your body. Be sure your hand is as close to you as possible. Do not put much weight on the hand; it is there to help you balance, *not* to lean on (see Figure 7.13).

5. Relax your shoulders, facial muscles and the inner thigh muscles and twist a bit further.

6. Check your body for tension and tightness. Mentally relax those parts that are keeping you from twisting further.

7. Take a breath, purse your lips, and blow it out. Twist a bit further, shifting your body away from the direction of the twist.

8. Hold the exercise for 30-60 seconds or until you are fatigued. Then return to a starting position by extending the back arm straight out from the shoulder, thumb up toward the ceiling, and sweeping the arm gently around and back to your lap.

9. Take two or three "Rock the Baby" breaths (p. 19), close your eyes, center and relax for a few seconds. Repeat the same movements on the left side. Repeat movements two more times.

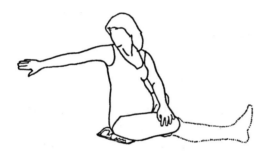

Figure 7.12   Going Into a Pregnancy Spinal Twist

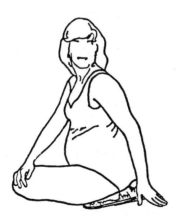

Figure 7.13   Pregnancy Spinal Twist

Cautions and Comments

- Once you have placed your hand on the mat in back of you, do not tip backwards. Move your hand closer to you for better balance.
- If you find that your hand falls asleep when placed on the floor behind you, move it up to your midback (see Figure 7.14).
- To increase the twist, you can bend your front arm and pull your front shoulder closer to the front opposite knee.

•Your upper back and chest should be doing most of the work during the twist, rather than your back arm and hand. Shift your consciousness to these areas and work them thoroughly.

•This exercise is an excellent preparation for labor, since you have to learn to relax *around* the stretch similar to the way you have to relax around your contractions. It takes time to learn to relax into this exercise, but its benefits will be increased if you take the necessary time.

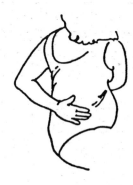

Figure 7.14   Midback Position for Pregnancy Spinal Twist

THE HEALTHY BACK SERIES

4a. Curl Back

Benefits

•Limbers up the spine and makes it flexible.
•Eliminates or minimizes pregnancy backache.
•Tones the central nervous system.
•Tones and tightens the thighs.
•Relieves neck strain.
•Strengthens the Rectus Abdominalis and iliopsoas muscle group.
•WARNING: *If you have separated recti muscles, do not do this exercise.* Instead, substitute the Pregnancy Curl-Up (page 79) and go on to the Bridge and the Lower Back Rocker.

Directions

1. Sitting with knees bent, feet flat, about 12"-16" apart, extend your arms straight out above the knees.

2. Take a deep breath and as you begin to exhale, move your upper body back so that the hands are above the knees and the lowest part of the back is rounded.

3. Exhale completely, blowing out in a curl-back position. When you run out of air, inhale as you come back into a sitting position (see Figure 7.15).

4. Repeat 5-10 times, coordinating exhalation with Curl Back and inhalation with return to start position. Make your movements smooth and graceful.

5. After 5-10 repetitions, ease onto your elbows (see Figure 7.15) and go into a flat back position.

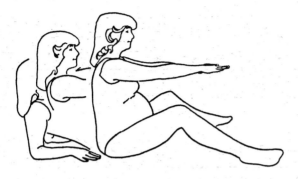

Figure 7.15 Curl Back

6. Take 3-4 "Rock the Baby" breaths (page 19) and rock your head from side to side to release tension in your neck.

Cautions and Comments

• This exercise *should not be practiced* by women with *separated recti muscles*. Have your caregiver check your recti muscles (abdominalis and linea alba) for a separation, or check yourself: 1. Lie on your back with your knees bent, tuck your chin to your chest, and raise your upper body about eight inches off the mat. 2. Gently press your fingertips into the center section of the abdomen from the breastbone to the pubic bone. If you notice a soft bulge in the middle abdominal area with two taut recti muscles on either side, this is an indication of a separation. 3. If your fingers can easily slide down into the abdomen and you feel no muscles blocking the way, there is a separation. Substitute the Pregnancy Half Curl-Up (page 80) for the Curl Back if you have a separation.

• When practicing Curl Backs, try to think of your abdominal recti muscles doing the work rather than your arms and shoulders.

• As the pregnancy progresses and this movement becomes more difficult to practice, place your hands on the sides of your legs and hold onto your outer thighs as you curl back.

• When you run out of breath, inhale and return to an upward sitting position.

• Remember to round the bottom of your back as you roll back.

• You may begin to shake slightly as you practice this exercise. This is perfectly normal, so keep practicing!

4b. Pregnancy Half Curl-Up

Benefits

• Aids maximum tone in the recti muscles and discourages further separation.

• Strengthens all of the abdominal muscle groups.

• Limbers up the spine and makes it flexible.

• Eliminates or minimizes pregnancy backache.

• Tones the central nervous system.

• Tones and tightens the thighs.

• Relieves neck strain.

Directions

1. Lying on your back, knees separated 12"-16" apart, cross your hands over your abdominal area so that as you raise your head, you will be able to support the two recti muscles.

2. Breathe in deeply. Then exhale and raise your head forward to your chest, gently pushing the separated stomach muscles towards each other (see Figure 7.16).

3. You should practice the Half Curl-Up to the point that you begin to feel a bulge.

4. Lower and repeat 3-5 times, twice a day.

Cautions and Comments

• The separation of your recti muscles is not a drastic situation. The hormones circulating in your body during pregnancy cause the central seam (linea alba) to soften and often separate. In addition, your stomach mus-

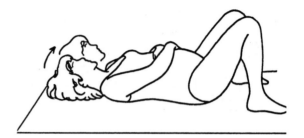

Figure 7.16 Pregnancy Half Curl-Up Position

cles are excessively stretched and strained during later pregnancy. A separation causes *no pain*, but you may suffer chronic backache throughout the pregnancy. You should always check on the status of your recti muscles. If and when you notice a separation, begin practicing the Pregnancy Half Curl-Up.

• You protect your recti muscles by holding them throughout this exercise.

4c. Pelvic Circles

Benefits

• Strengthen and stretch the rectus and oblique abdominalis groups, the erector spinae (middle and lower postvertebrals), the gluteal muscle group, the hamstrings (biceps femoris).

• Limber up the spine and make it flexible.

• Eliminate or minimize pregnancy backache.

• Tone the central nervous system.
• Tone and tighten the thighs.
• Relieve neck strain.

Directions

1. In a flat back position, with your arms at your sides, check to see that your feet are hip distance apart and facing forward or even a bit inward.

2. Shift your awareness to the waist area of your back and flatten it to the mat.

3. Now shift your awareness and your weight to the right hip and allow your legs to fall over a bit to the right.

4. Flatten the coccyx (lowest part of the spine) onto the mat and feel the waist area arch up slightly.

5. Shift your weight over to your left hip area and allow the legs to fall slightly to the left.

6. Having touched all four quadrants of your circle, come back to the waist area and imagine that you are drawing a smooth circle with your lower back. Feel your body slightly touching the mat as it draws the circle on the mat. Let your legs flow with the movement of the lower back as it makes a wide, slow circle.

7. Circle five times in each direction, making the widest circle you can. Breathe normally throughout the movement (see Figure 7.17). Feel your lower back warming, stretching and tingling. Then immediately go on to the Bridge.

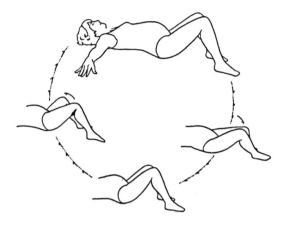

Figure 7.17 Pelvic Circles

Cautions and Comments

- Pelvic Circles beautifully prepare your lower back for the Bridge.
- Try to make your circles as even as possible. Close your eyes and tune into the motion in your pelvis.
- Your baby may particularly like this movement, for it is getting a free ride!

4d. The Bridge

Benefits

- Strengthens the cervical, thoracic, and lumbar postvertebrals (erector spinae), rectus abdominalis, gluteus maximus, the biceps femoris, the soleus.
- Stretches the middle and the lower (erector spinae) postvertebrals, the iliopsoas muscle group, the rectus fe-moris, the pectoralis major.
- Limbers up the spine and makes it flexible.
- Eliminates or minimizes pregnancy backache.
- Tones the central nervous system.
- Tones and tightens the thighs.
- Relieves neck strain.

Directions

1. Check to see that your arms are at your sides, your legs are hip distance apart, feet separated and facing forward as you flatten the waist area to the mat and tighten your buttocks.

2. Imagine that there is a rope secured around the baby area lifting the middle section of your body up into the air. Lift high enough so that there is a straight line between your shoulders and buttocks. Shift up a bit higher for added stretch to the thighs but not high enough to overarch your back (see Figure 7.18).

3. While holding this Bridge, lift your toes so that the balls of the feet are off the floor and you are working your shin muscles to prevent leg cramps in the calves. Hold for thirty seconds and flatten feet.

4. Breathe normally, keeping your awareness on how your body feels holding this pose. Keep the buttocks tight as you hold the Bridge for as long as is comfortable.

5. When coming out of the Bridge, imagine that your spine is a pearl necklace. Extend your arms straight out from the shoulders, then begin to lower the small vertebraes (or pearls) one at a time—first in your neck, then in the upper back, then in the middle of the back, and finally in the lower back.

6. Take 1-2 minutes for the descent. Close your eyes and feel each pearl (vertebrae) touching the mat.

7. When you return to your starting position, move your head from side to side to release tension in your neck and take 1-2 "Rock the Baby" breaths (see p. 19). Then immediately go on to the Lower Back Rocker.

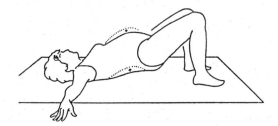

Figure 7.18   The Bridge Position

Cautions and Comments

- You may find it helpful, if you have a particularly weak back, to place your hands on the back of your waist, elbows bent and on the mat during the elevated segment of the Bridge. As your thighs and back strengthen, you will no longer have to do this.
- The Bridge exercise has been used by many caregivers to help turn breech babies. A breech baby lies in the uterus with feet facing the cervix. It doesn't work *all* the time, however.
- You can also practice the Bridge by placing straight legs on your bed and then proceeding to lift up the baby area. Remember to flatten the waist area and tighten the buttocks before lifting up.
- Try twisting your hips from side to side while you are lifted into a Bridge to strengthen your buttocks and work your abdomen.

•For increased stretching in the calves and soleus muscles, you can go onto your toes when up into the Bridge pose. However, if you are prone to calf cramps, *do not* practice this variation, for it may cause more cramps to develop. Instead, practice Direction #4 of the Bridge.

4e. Lower Back Rocker

Benefits

•Stretches the back (erector spinae) postvertebrals, gluteus maximus, and the gluteus medius.
•Strengthens the abdominal muscle groups.
•Limbers up the spine and makes it flexible.
•Eliminates or minimizes pregnancy backache.
•Tones the central nervous system.
•Tones and tightens the thighs.
•Relieves neck strain.

Directions

1. Immediately following your descent and breaths, bring each knee on either side of the baby, place your hands below your knees and gently rock side to side to massage the lower back (see Figure 7.19).

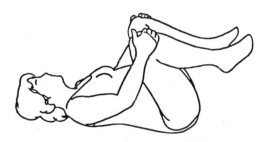

Figure 7.19 Lower Back Rocker

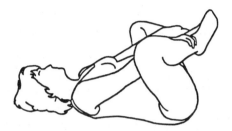

Figure 7.20 Lower Back Rocker With Knees Extended

2. A variation on Lower Back Rocker, which really massages the sacrum and coccyx area, is practiced by placing the soles of your feet together, knees out to the side and hands on ankles. Gently rock side to side in this position (see Figure 7.20).

3. After rocking for 1-2 minutes, shift your body onto the right side. Take 1-2 "Rock the Baby" breaths (p. 19), close your eyes, tune in and center as you relax for a few seconds.

Cautions and Comments

•Many pregnant women love this series because it releases lower back muscular tension and eliminates chronic pain.
•The Pelvic Circles, Bridge, and Lower Back Rocker should be practiced all together, one right after the other.

5. Side Leg Circles with a Half Bow

Benefits

- Strengthen the rectus and oblique abdominalis group, the latissimus dorsi, the deltoideus, the upper trapezius, the bicep brachii, the iliopsoas, the rectus femoris muscles.
- Stretch the latissimus dorsi, gluteus medius, the hamstring muscle group, and the gastrocnemius-soleus muscle group.
- Loosen the entire pelvic area.
- Help to reduce postural edema in the legs by draining excess blood out of tired legs.
- Help relieve lower backache.
- Tone and keep legs shapely.
- Firm the arms and strengthen the shoulders.
- Often, the Half Bow will help to relieve lower groin cramps.

Directions for Leg Circle

1. Lie on your right side, legs together, with your right hand on your right ear. Make your body into a straight line (see Figure 7.21).

2. Once you are straight, bend your bottom leg for better balance. Bend the top leg facing the top knee toward the ceiling. Straighten the leg up into the air, clasping the ankle with your top hand.

3. Hold the stretch for 10-30 seconds. Be aware of your calf and thigh muscles stretching. Keep breathing normally. Check your facial muscles for tension. Release your jaw muscles by slightly separating your teeth.

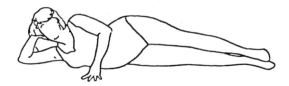

Figure 7.21 Getting Your Body Straight for Practicing Leg Circles

4. Circle your elevated foot at the ankle, 5-10 times in each direction. Wiggle your toes and feel the warmth in your foot (see Figure 7.22).

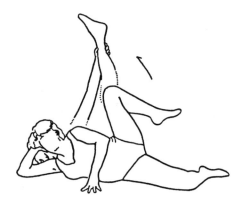

Figure 7.22 Thigh Stretch Position

5. Imagine that there is a wall directly behind you, so that when you begin to move your entire leg in a circle, it cannot go behind you. Begin to make circles in the air using your entire leg. Keep your awareness on the warming

and loosening of your top hip joint as the leg circles. Make 5-10 circles in each direction (see Figure 7.23).

6. When the leg becomes tired, lower it and bring it down in front of the bent lower leg. Take one or two "Rock the Baby" breaths (p. 19) and relax.

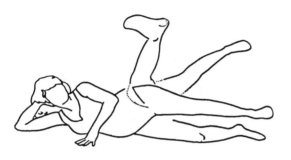

Figure 7.23   Leg Circles on the Side

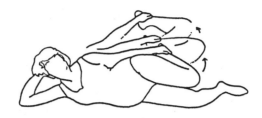

Figure 7.24   The Half Bow

Directions for Half Bow

1. Bend the top leg, and reach back and grab your top ankle using your top hand (see Figure 7.24).

2. Pull the top bent leg *straight* back, tipping the top hip bone and chest so that they face down toward the mat. Make sure the bottom leg is bent for better balance.

3. Gently raise the top foot up toward the ceiling, keeping your top arm straight. You should feel a stretch throughout your top arm and leg and across your back (see Figure 7.24).

4. Hold the Half Bow exercise for 15-30 seconds or as long as is comfortable and then lower.

5. Bring the top knee next to the top shoulder and wrap your top arm around the top of your leg. Hold for a few seconds and release.

6. Take one or two "Rock the Baby" breaths (p. 19) and relax for a few seconds. Close your eyes, look inside, check the body for tension, then let it go.

7. Roll over and do both movements on the other side, or practice some Baby Curls (p. 86) and then practice on second side.

Cautions and Comments

- When making leg circles, start with small ones but finish with the largest circles you can make. This is very important for keeping the pelvic area loose and moveable in preparation for the birthing process.
- When practicing the Half Bow, be sure to keep your top arm straight for maximum stretch. If you feel a tight pull across your abdomen, lower the top bent leg a bit to minimize the pull.
- Some women prefer to practice these two exercises with their heads resting on a flat lower arm. See which way is more comfortable for you.
- During the later months when your legs become increasingly heavy, you may find doing leg circles to be quite

uncomfortable. Instead, bend your top leg and pretend you are riding a bicycle with that leg. In essence you are drawing a circle in the air with your knee. Make 5-10 circles and

then reverse direction.

•In the last trimester of pregnancy, the hip joints often become very sensitive. You may have to reduce the number of leg circles you practice.

6. Baby Curls

Benefits

•Strengthen the internal and external oblique abdominalis muscle groups.
•Stretch the lower lumbar spine postvertebrals (erector spinae).
•Prepare the oblique abdominalis muscle group for the pushing stage of labor.
•Gently strengthen your lower back, arms and shoulders.
•Keep your buttocks tight and firm.
•Help build your confidence because Baby Curls are a challenge.

Directions for Variation I

1. In a back-lying position, with the knees bent and the feet hip distance apart facing forward or inward, extend your arms above the chest, placing your right hand on left elbow and left hand on right elbow (see Figure 7.25).

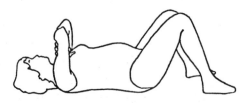

Figure 7.25 Getting Ready for Baby Curls

2. Inhale and then roll the upper part of your body over to the edge of your right shoulder.

3. Exhale, blowing out of your mouth, and use the power of the exhalation to lift your head and shoulders a small distance off the mat. Aim the middle of your arms toward the opposite knee (see Figure 7.26).

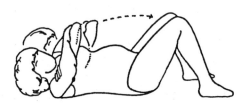

Figure 7.26 Baby Curl Position

4. When you run out of air, lower your upper body and smoothly inhale, as you roll over to the edge of the left shoulder. Using the exhalation, lift your upper body, aim the middle of the arms toward the left knee, and blow out. When out of air, inhale and lower down.

5. Repeat 5-10 times on each side, keeping your lower back and buttocks on

the mat and remembering to *exhale* when you *lift* and *inhale* when you *lower*.

6. Keep your consciousness on your abdominal oblique muscles located on either side of the rib cage and abdomen.

7. When you have finished a comfortable number of Baby Curls, bring your arms down to your sides, and rock your head from side to side to release any tightness and tension in the neck and shoulders. Roll over onto your side and take two or three "Rock the Baby" breaths (see p. 19), close your eyes, tune in, center and relax for a few seconds.

Directions for Variation II

1. Lie on your back with a pillow under your head and upper back—knees bent, hip distance apart, feet facing forward or inward.

2. Extend your arms up into the air above your chest, with your palms together (see Figure 7.27).

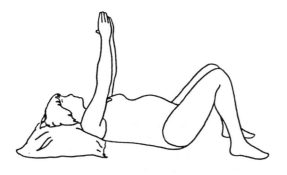

Figure 7.27 Getting Ready for Baby Curls—Variation II

3. Inhale and roll over to the edge of the right shoulder.

4. Lift the upper body up as you exhale, blowing out of your mouth. Stretch your hands out as close to the right knee as possible (see Figure 7.28).

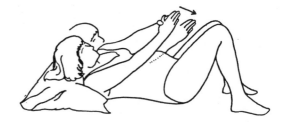

Figure 7.28 Baby Curl Position—Variation II

5. When you run out of air, lower and inhale as you roll over to the edge of the left shoulder, reach your hands toward the left knee, and blow out.

6. Repeat 5-10 times on each side, coordinating your breath with your movement.

7. Roll over onto your side, take two or three "Rock the Baby" breaths (see p. 19), close your eyes, tune in, center, see what the baby is doing, and relax for a few seconds.

Cautions and Comments

• Coordinate your breath with each movement during Baby Curls. *Do not hold your breath!*

• Variation I of Baby Curls is easier. Move on to Variation II when you find it comfortable to do Variation I ten times or more on each side.

• A more difficult version of Baby Curls can be practiced by placing both hands, palms down, loosely on the back of your head, with elbows out to the side. Inhale and roll over to the edge of the right shoulder and lift the upper body up toward the opposite knee while exhaling through pursed lips. Try to keep your arms straight out on either side of your head, rather than moving forward. Practice 5-10 times on each side, co-ordinating your breath with each movement (see Figure 7.29).

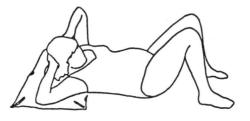

Figure 7.29 Difficult Version of Baby Curls

•This exercise may grow progressively more difficult as the end of pregnancy nears. You can cut down on the number of repetitions you practice, but do not stop practicing.

•As you lift the upper body, be sure you feel the oblique abdominalis muscle groups working on the opposite side of the body. If you do not feel the muscles working, try a slightly different angle to the side until you feel the abdominals working. You should *not* be straining your neck muscles.

•When practicing Variation II, do not lift your upper body with your arms and neck; use your abdominals.

•As you push your baby into our world and your body is put to the test, you will personally experience the dividends of this exercise.

7. Pelvic Floor Toners

ANAL LOCK

Benefits

•Strengthen the levatores ani, coccygeus, sphincter ani externus, bulbosprongiosus, tranversus perinei super-facialis and sphincter urethrae (all part of the perianal and perineal muscle group).

•Massage and tone the female sex organs.

•Are highly beneficial for the nerves and organs of the reproductive system.

•Help prevent constipation and hemorrhoids.

•Keep your sexual area responsive while preparing the birth canal area for your baby's birth.

Directions

1. In a side-lying position, close your eyes and become aware of your breath. Inhale and exhale smoothly (see Figure 7.30).

2. Inhale again, this time contracting your buttocks muscles—feel your anal

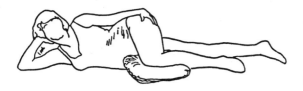

Figure 7.30 Anal Lock Position

muscles, vaginal muscles, and urethral muscles contracting.

3. Exhale, with your eyes closed, and
    feel the release and opening of the
    birth canal. Connect with that open-
    ing feeling, for you will experience it
    during the birthing process.

4. Repeat the Anal Lock 5-10 times.

5. Take one or two "Rock the Baby"
    breaths (see p. 19) and relax for a few
    seconds.

Cautions and Comments

•With some practice you can learn to
release and contract only the anal
muscles, only the vaginal muscles,
and only the urethral muscles. This,
however, takes time and effort.
•Practice this exercise when you are at
work, two or three times a day.
•This exercise should be practiced
right after the birth of your baby, to
help promote quick healing of the
birth canal and episiotomy (if you
have one).

PELVIC FLOOR EXERCISES (KEGELS)

Benefits

•Strengthen the pelvic floor (bulbospongiosus, transverse perinei superficialis and profundus, the
sphincter urethrae and ischiocavernosus), thereby giving better support to your growing uterus and
baby.
•Prevent trickling urine while laughing, coughing, etc.
•Help prevent damage to the birth canal during the birth of your baby.
•Help relieve pelvic congestion or
swelling during pregnancy.

Directions

1. The next time you go into the bath-
    room to urinate, separate your legs
    and stop the flow of urine after only
    half of it is passed.

2. Close your eyes and feel the con-
    tracted pelvic floor muscles.

3. Urinate a bit more and then contract
    again.

4. Contract your pelvic floor muscles
    four to five times until you are totally
    familiar with how these muscles feel
    contracted and relaxed.

5. During your practice session of the
    "Basic Nine," in a side-lying position,
    place your fingertips right above your
    pubic bone, contract your pelvic floor
    muscles and hold for two seconds.
    Release the muscles and repeat ten
    more times.

6. Practice up to fifty a day, in five sets of
    ten.

Cautions and Comments

- Overexercising the pelvic floor muscles will tire them out, so don't overdo it.
- Many people refer to these exercises as Kegels (named after the doctor who first made them popular) or ex-

ercises. Once you strengthen and tone the pelvic floor, you will find that your sexual pleasure will increase. Your partner can check your tone while you are making love. The tighter the muscles, the higher the pleasure quotient.

8. Chest Expansion or Support for the "Milk Factory"

Benefits

- Stretches the hamstring muscle group, gastronemius-soleus muscle group, the gluteus maximus, the pectoralis major, the shoulder rotator cuff muscle group, the gastrocnemius-soleus muscle group.
- Strengthens the upper thigh (quadraceps muscle group), lower back (lumbar region), postvertebrals (erector spinae), the rhomboideus, the middle and lower trapezius muscles.
- Releases tension and tightness in the neck, shoulders, upper and lower back while strengthening these areas.
- Develops and strengthens the pectoralis muscle group supporting the breasts.
- Tones, shapes and tightens the thighs.
- Is a quick energizer.
- Expands the lung and chest area for increased breathing capacity.

Directions

1. From a side-lying position, use your hands and arms to walk your upper body into a sitting position (see Figure 7.31). Bend one leg, placing one foot on the mat. Shift your hands so they are on the mat, palms on the floor between your legs. Shift your other leg into a squat position (see Figure 7.32).

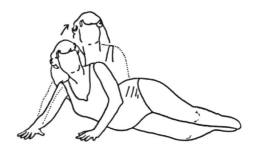

Figure 7.31 Walking Yourself Into a Sitting-Up Position

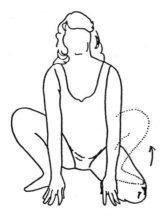

Figure 7.32 Getting Into a Squatting Position

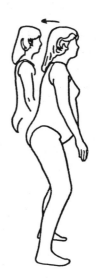

Figure 7.34 Shifting Your Feet So That They Face Forward

2. Make sure your feet are on a 45° angle out to the sides, as you push down on your hands. Keep your chin up and slowly begin to lift up into the air (see Figure 7.33).

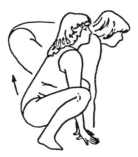

Figure 7.33 Pushing Out of a Squatting Position

3. Halfway up, shift your feet so that they are facing forward, thereby taking any strain off your knees. Continue to unroll slowly up into a standing position (see Figure 7.34).

4. Once you are comfortably standing, take one or two "Rock the Baby" breaths (see p. 19).

5. Move your feet so they are at least three feet apart, on a 45° angle out to the sides. Tuck your buttocks under and feel yourself straightening up and getting taller.

6. Clasp your hands behind you, palms facing up toward your head. Inhale and gently raise the clasped hands up; exhale and lower the hands back down to your buttocks. Repeat this movement 3-4 times to warm and limber the pectoral muscles (see Figure 7.35).

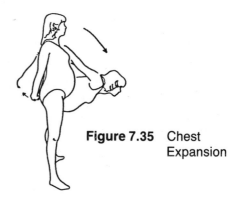

Figure 7.35 Chest Expansion

7. Contract your pelvic floor muscles. When the shoulders feel warm, slowly bend forward from the bottom of your buttocks, so that your upper body is parallel to the floor. Keep your knees slightly bent and unlocked. Keep your hands near your buttocks as you go forward. When you are in a comfortable forward-bend position with your chin up, slowly inhale and raise the arms up as high as is comfortable (see Figure 7.36). Hold for 30-60 seconds, breathing normally.

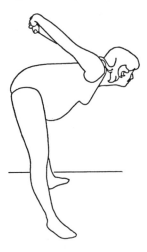

Figure 7.36   Chest Expansion Bending Forward

8. With your chin up, slowly begin to unroll upward back into a standing position. When you are upright, take 1-2 "Rock the Baby" breaths (see p. 19).

9. With your hands still clasped behind you, turn your right foot on a 90° angle to the right and move the left foot inward on a 45° angle to the right. Now move your upper body so that it is centered over the right leg.

10. Slowly lower the upper body as close to the right knee as possible. Inhale, then exhale and raise your arms up as high as you can. Hold this posture for 15-30 seconds, breathing normally. If this is painful, bend the knee in the position shown in Figure 7.37.

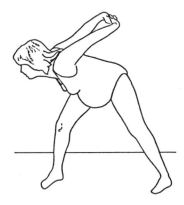

Figure 7.37   Chest Expansion to the Side

11. Keeping your upper body parallel to the mat, slowly shift it over to the left side, after shifting your left foot to a 90° angle to the side and the right foot to a 45° angle toward the left.

12. Move your body back to the center and inhale. Then exhale as you raise the arms up even higher in a clasped position. You will be surprised to discover that they will reach quite a bit higher!

13. Imagine that there is a rope around your hands slowly pulling you up into a standing position. Once you are fully upright, take one or two "Rock the Baby" breaths (see p. 19). Close your eyes, look inward, and see how you and your baby feel as you relax for a few seconds.

Cautions and Comments

- •This exercise stretches many sets of muscles in your chest and back in ways they are not used to. So you may find some resistance to these movements when you first begin to practice. Keep working and you will notice your upper body opening up and becoming freer and looser as your lower body becomes firmer.
- •It is very important to remember to move each foot to a 90° angle to the side, with the second foot on a 45° angle facing the 90° foot. By placing the feet correctly in the side stretch movements of Chest Expansion, you align the leg and foot for proper stretch and prevent injury.

- •It is a good idea to practice this exercise next to a chair at first, for you have to develop your concentration skills to balance correctly in the movements to the side.
- •To increase the stretch across your chest and shoulders, try some of the clasped hand movements with your palms touching and thumbs together.
- •After you have practiced Chest Expansion for a while, you may want to combine the forward bending movements with the side stretching movements. Decide what feels best for you.

9. Complete Relaxation

Benefits

- •Releases tension by deeply relaxing the muscles and the nervous system.
- •Trains you to be able to completely relax at will.
- •Restores peace of mind.

- •Can contribute to a shorter labor.
- •Deepens your conscious connections with your future baby.

(For complete directions, turn to Chapter 8).

SALUTE TO THE CHILD

The "Salute to the Child," an innovative concept in prenatal exercise, evolved quite naturally from a number of highly beneficial and safe exercises which can be practiced throughout pregnancy. By incorporating these interwoven exercises into your daily routine, you should continue to feel limber and energetic during the entire nine months. "Salute to the Child" will prepare your body both physically and mentally for the birth experience. During each exercise, first feel the particular stretches; second, focus in on your future child for a few seconds; then go on to the next position. Note that some positions require more deep breathing during rest intervals than others.

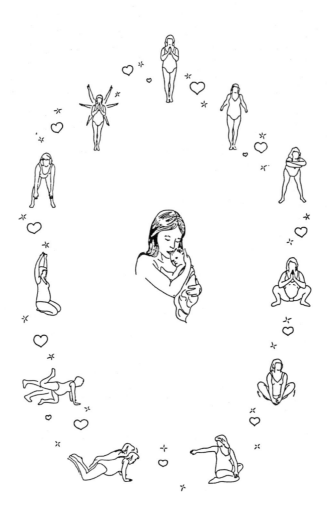

Salute to the Child

Benefits

- Prepares the appropriate muscle groups for the rigors of birth.
- Keeps your spine and body flexible and supple.
- Develops your concentration skills.
- Preserves and tones those parts of your body that are not directly affected by the pregnancy.
- Helps to foster a more direct relationship between you and your baby.
- Releases tension; produces a heightened feeling of peace and relaxation.

Directions for Position 1: Welcome Pose

1. Stand up straight with your feet as close together as is comfortable. Spread out your toes and imagine that you have long roots extending down from your toes, going deep into the earth. These roots keep you anchored and balanced.

2. Place your hands (palms together) next to your breast bone. Take one or two "Rock the Baby" breaths (see p. 19) as you become centered. As you inhale, let tranquility and stillness envelop you; as you exhale, release any nervousness and fatigue (see Figure 7.38).

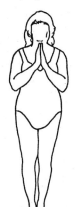

Figure 7.38 Welcome Pose

Directions for Position 2: Shoulderblade Stretch

1. Stretch your arms directly out in front of you, palms together, while you focus on the stretching feeling across your shoulders and upper back (see Figure 7.39).

2. Twist your arms so that the palms face outward (see Figure 7.40). Hold for five seconds, then bring your arms behind you, shoulder distance apart (see Figure 7.41).

3. Arch your chest and the baby area forward as you gently push your shoulder blades together. Hold this position for 5-10 seconds, breathing normally.

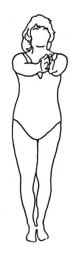

Figure 7.39 Shoulderblade Stretch in Front

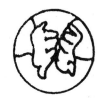

Figure 7.40 Arm Twist

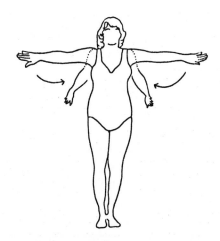

Figure 7.41 Shoulderblade Stretch in Back

Directions for Position 3: Cradle Stretch

1. Release your arms and bring them slowly forward until they are finally in front of your chest. Place your right hand on the left elbow and the left hand on the right elbow (see Figure 7.42).

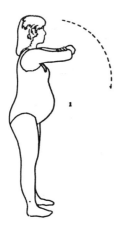

Figure 7.42   Going Into a Cradle Stretch

2. As your arms move forward, spread your legs so that they are three feet apart and on a 45° angle facing outward. Make sure that your back is straight and you are standing tall when your hands go into the cradle position.

3. Stretch your arms forward in this position, keeping your back straight and bending from your buttocks as far down as you can without losing the "stretch" feeling in your shoulders and upper arms. Hold for 5-10 seconds, breathing normally.

4. Holding your arms in the cradle position, turn as far to the right as you can. Hold, breathing normally for 5-10 sec-

onds (see Figure 7.43). Keep your knees loose and unlocked.

5. Repeat this movement on the left side, holding for 5-10 seconds and breathing normally.

6. Repeat the movements side to side, trying to be as graceful as you can and pretending you are holding and rocking your baby in your arms.

7. Return to center, letting your arms drop down to your sides. Take one or two "Rock the Baby" breaths (see page 19).

8. Be *aware* of your posture: shoulders back and down, chin up, buttocks tucked under. Take a breath down to your child. Inhale energy directly to the child. Exhale, opening your mouth wide and just letting it go.

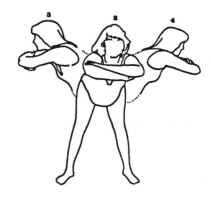

Figure 7.43   Stretching to Either Side

Directions for Position 4: Squat with Baby Breath

1. Allow your hands to gently rise in front of you, keeping palms down and arms straight out in front of you. Slowly bend your knees and feel yourself going down into a squat (see Figures 7.44 and 7.45). NOTE: *If you have varicose veins, please do not do this movement.*

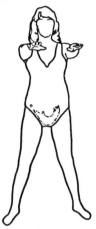

Figure 7.44   Starting Into a Squat

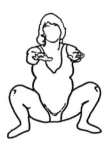

Figure 7.45   Squatting Pose

2. Once you've gone down into a squat, place your hands in front of you on the mat for balance. You'll want to separate your feet a bit more, and try to get your feet flat (if you can).

3. Place your right elbow on your right knee, left elbow on the left knee. Put the palms together, with fingertips pointing upward (see Figure 7.46).

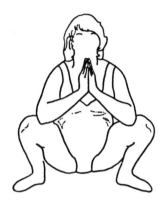

Figure 7.46   Position for Practicing "Baby Breath"

4. Use your imagination. Inhale, imagining that the air is going directly to your child through your navel. As you exhale, open your mouth wide and say "Ahh."

5. Again, inhale directly to the baby. When you exhale, imagine that the air is coming out of your birth canal and make the "Ahh" sound again.

6. Feel a slight "pushing down" in the birth canal area. Inhale once more. Exhale and push gently. NOTE: *This is a very subtle movement. Feel it on the inside of your pelvic floor.*

Directions for Position 5: Butterfly

1. Let your hands come down behind you on the mat. Slowly lower your buttocks (see Figure 7.47).

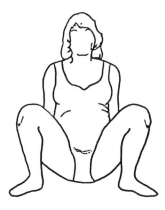

Figure 7.47   Coming Out of the Squat

2. Place the soles of your feet together. Place one hand on each ankle. Slowly raise your knees up toward your chest as you inhale (see Figure 7.48).

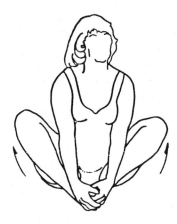

Figure 7.48   Butterfly with Knees Raised

3. Now exhale, pulling your head down as close to your toes as you can without getting out of breath or feeling pain (see Figure 7.49).

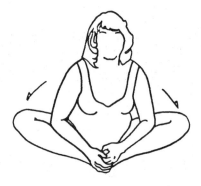

Figure 7.49   Butterfly with Knees Lowered

4. Inhale as you come up slowly, bringing your knees up. Exhale while coming forward, with your elbows on the outside of the legs.

5. Inhale again as you come up, bringing your knees up. Exhale while coming forward. This time bring your head down as close to your toes as you can. Keep breathing normally (see Figure 7.50).

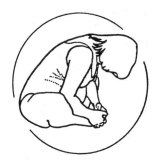

Figure 7.50   Forward Bend

6. Stretch a little further, feeling the inner thigh stretching. Notice how it feels. Hold for a little bit longer and then unroll slowly, coming back up.

Directions for Position 6: Spinal Twist in a "Z"

1. Clasp your hands together, placing them on your right knee (see Figure 7.51). Gently roll the right knee so that it is next to your left foot (see Figure 7.52). The left foot should be right in the middle of your body. Your right heel should be near your right hip. Your legs look like the letter "Z."

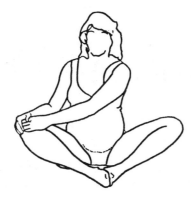

Figure 7.51 Shifting Into a "Z" Sitting Position

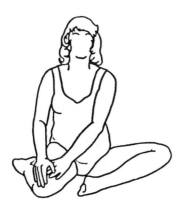

Figure 7.52 "Z" Sitting Position

2. Keep your left hand on your right knee. Extend your right arm straight out from your shoulder. Sit up a little straighter.

3. Point your right pinky up toward the ceiling. Have the fingers of the right hand remain flat. Push back behind you, looking at your hand as you push (see Figure 7.53).

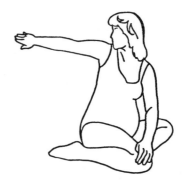

Figure 7.53 Hand Placement for Spinal Twist in a "Z" Sitting Position

4. Make sure your head is up straight. Keep breathing normally. Bend the front arm. Push a little further back behind you. Feel a good stretch in the middle of your back.

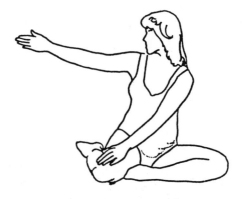

Figure 7.54 Thumb-Up Position for Spinal Twist in a "Z" Sitting Position

5. Slowly sweeping the back arm around, thumb up toward the ceiling, gracefully bring it back in front of you (see Figure 7.54).

6. Repeat this same motion on the other side.

7. Release the second back arm and gently swing it around, back to the front. Do this slowly and gracefully. Bring your hands down to your lap.

8. Inhale and take the breath down to your child. Exhale and rock your baby back.

Directions for Position 7: Pregnancy Push-Up

1. Slide your hands down your thighs and onto the mat (see Figure 7.55). Shift your body onto all fours. Remain on your hands and knees (see Figure 7.56).

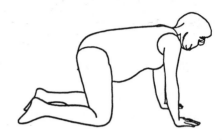

Figure 7.56   Hands and Knees Position

2. Separate your hands so that they are shoulder distance apart, fingers forward *or* facing each other.

3. Move your knees back about eight inches. Lift your feet up off the mat. Cross your feet at the ankles. You should now be leaning on your hands and knees.

4. Be sure that your back is perfectly straight and flat. Drop the hips a little bit.

5. Take a breath. As you exhale, lower your body *half way* toward the mat. Inhale and come back up (see Figure 7.57).

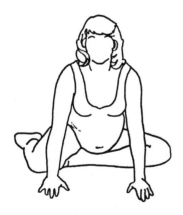

Figure 7.55   Getting on All Fours

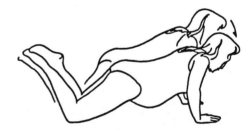

Figure 7.57   Pregnancy Push-Up

6. Work at your own pace and do 5-10 Pregnancy Push-Ups. Remember to exhale when you do the work of lowering. Inhale as you come up.

Directions for Position 8: Rainbow Stretches

1. Separate your feet and place them flat on the mat.

2. Separate your knees. Stretch the buttocks back onto your heels.

3. Let your head come down on the mat right in front of your body. Keep your arms extended straight out. Stretch your arms and just relax.

4. Take a moment or two to take a breath into the baby and your body. Now let it go. Feel the shoulders and arms relaxing (see Figure 7.58).

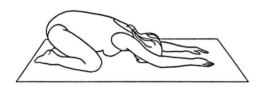

Figure 7.58 Relaxing Rainbow Stretch

5. Shift position, moving your knees underneath your hips and your hands underneath your shoulders. Shift into an "all fours" position.

6. Keep your head up in this flat-back position. Take a breath. As you exhale, hug your baby close to your body. Let it go.

7. Arch your back up toward the ceiling. Feel it being stretched (see Figure 7.59). Continue breathing, keeping your chin up. Maximize your stretch and then flatten out.

8. Repeat this movement several times. Take a breath down to the child, and let it go.

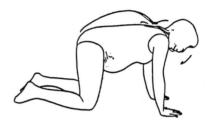

Figure 7.59 Exerting Rainbow Stretch

Directions for Position 9: Leg Stretch on All Fours

1. Shift all your weight onto your left leg. Bring the right knee up into the air. Feel the right thigh being stretched (see Figure 7.60).

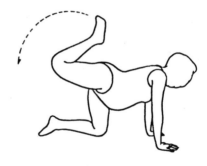

Figure 7.60 Leg Stretch with a Bent Knee

2. Straighten the right leg out in the air behind you. Flex your foot and feel the entire leg stretch.

3. Place the right foot down on the mat. Try to get your right heel as close to the mat as you can, with your toes on the mat. Feel the stretch all the way

from your buttocks down to your heel on the right side (see Figure 7.61).

4. If you choose, you can look through your legs toward your feet, or turn your head, stretching your neck. But always look toward that right foot.

5. Releasing, bring your right knee back up into the air. Push it up as high as you can without overarching your back. Feel the groin area being stretched. Then allow the knee to come down on the mat.

6. Take a breath and let it go.

7. Repeat these same movements on the other side. NOTE: *During the last two or three months of your pregnancy, you may want to sit back on your heels in the Zen Sitting Position and take 1-5 deep breaths before proceeding to the second leg.*

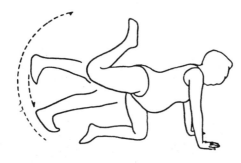

Figure 7.61   Leg Stretch with the Toes Curled Under

Directions for Position 10: Arm Stretching in the Zen Position

1. Slowly shift back onto your heels, placing your buttocks directly on your heels and feet.

2. You should find yourself sitting upright. Put your head up a little straighter. Check your jaw muscles, letting these muscles relax (see Figure 7.62).

3. Take a breath to the baby and let it go.

4. Gently allow your arms to float up into the air above your head.

5. Clasp your hands together, palms up toward the ceiling. Keep your arms nice and straight.

6. Feel the stretch on either side of your body, as you begin to move over to the right side. Keep the buttocks steady as you stretch the upper body over to the right side (see Figure 7.63).

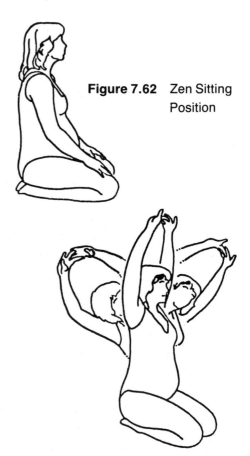

Figure 7.62   Zen Sitting Position

Figure 7.63   Arm Stretches in the Zen Sitting Position

7. Now return to center and go over to the left side. Tune in and see how it feels.

8. Come back to the center and go over to the right side again. Then, go again to the center and over to the left side.

9. Bring your arms straight up above your head. Push your hands back. Feel the stretch in your upper back and neck.

10. Gently lower your clasped hands, bringing them down directly onto the baby area (see Figure 7.64). Take a breath to the baby. Make the "Ahh" sound as you let it go.

11. In the late stages of your pregnancy, you can clasp your elbows above your head and move from side to side (see Figure 7.64a).

Figure 7.64 Breathing to the Baby

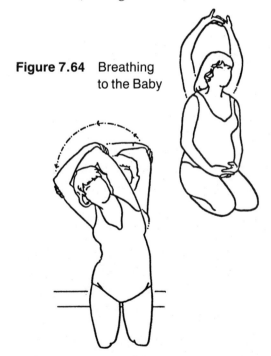

Figure 7.64a Stretching to the Side During the Later Months

Directions for Position 11: Stretching Out of Squat

1. Separating your knees, place your hands on the mat directly in front of you, with palms down and fingers facing forward.

2. Place one foot flat on the mat. Shift your weight over onto that foot and then gently place the other foot flat on the mat. You are now in a squat position (see Figure 7.65).

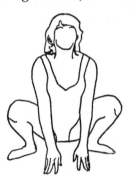

Figure 7.65 Stretching Out of the Squat

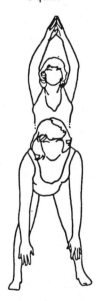

Figure 7.66 Turning Your Feet Halfway Out of the Squat

3. Keep your chin up. As you push down on the mat, slowly begin to straighten up.

4. Half-way up, turn your feet so that they face directly forward (see Figure 7.66). Feel your back unrolling one little vertebra at a time.

Directions for Position 12: Heaven/Earth Stretch

1. Keep your head and chin up. Your fingertips should now be touching right in front of your body (see Figure 7.67).

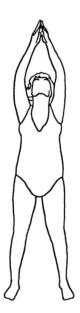

Figure 7.67   Head and Chin Up in the Heaven/Earth Stretch

2. Stretch the fingertips up toward the heavens—way, way up!

3. Now separate your hands, turning them palms down. Sweep the arms down gently on either side and finish

with the palms right in front of you (see Figure 7.68).

4. Place your feet together. Take 1-2 "Rock the Baby" breaths (see page 19) and repeat this series 1-3 times. Follow with a Complete Relaxation (see page 158) for 10-20 minutes.

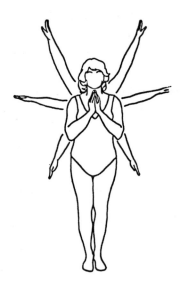

Figure 7.68   Sweeping the Palms Down

Cautions and Comments

- This series should be devoted entirely to your baby and to developing gracefulness, flexibility and strength in your own body.
- Do not be overwhelmed by the number of different movements contained in this series. Once you become familiar with them, you will probably discover some favorite positions. But don't leave out those movements that you dislike. Each movement in the series is beautifully utilitarian for the pregnant woman, so hang in there!

• In the early and later months of your pregnancy, you may experience some dizziness when coming out of the squat. Do not be alarmed. If this happens, shift your body onto your knees in a kneeling position, keeping the rest of your body straight, and proceed with the described arm movements.

• Some women find the Zen sitting position uncomfortable. Try shifting the legs to the side instead.

• As you practice this series, try to increase the number of seconds that each position is held. *You should never exceed thirty seconds in any one position.*

• Try to include one "Salute to the Child" series in every practice session.

STANDING EXERCISES

Your legs may tire and swell more easily during pregnancy; the following exercises and postures will help to invigorate them. Remember to practice a variety of postures during each practice session. Add one or two of the following postures to your daily routine. Try each posture at least once to get a feel for it.

The Back Stretcher

Benefits

• Stretches the entire body.
• Tones the arms, back, thighs and calves.
• Strengthens and tones all portions of the trapezii muscles, the rhomboideus muscle group, the cervical and thoracic postvertebrals (erector spinae), the deltoideus muscle groups, and the triceps brachii muscles.
• Stretches the gastrocnemius-soleus muscle complex, the gluteus maximus, the lumbar spine postvertebrals (erector spinae), the pectoralis muscles, the latissimus dorsi, and the anterior chest wall fascia.

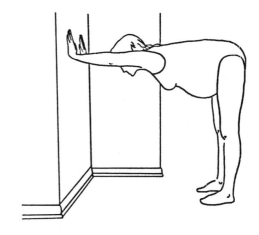

Figure 7.69 The Back Stretcher

Directions

1. Stand directly in front of a wall. Place your hands on the wall, shoulder distance apart. Walk away from the wall until you begin to feel a stretch in your back, arms and thighs (see Figure 7.69).

2. Feel a terrific stretch in your arms and shoulders as well as in your thighs. Hold the stretch for thirty seconds to two minutes.

3. Slowly walk toward the wall as you raise your head first and then your body.

4. Take 2-3 "Rock the Baby" breaths (see page 19) and repeat the exercise two more times.

Cautions and Comments

- This is a terrific stretch to do in the shower after you have turned the water off.
- Try to get your heels down as close to the ground as possible. When you have succeeded, move your legs back half an inch and try it again.
- If facing downward makes you dizzy, try keeping your head up.

Hip Rotator

Benefits

- Stretches all lumbo-pelvic-femoral muscle groups attached to the pelvis from the femur or from the lumbar spinae, including the gluteals, hip adductors, piriformis, multifidus, iliolumbar fascia, iliopsoas and perineal muscles (pelvic floor).
- Relieves tired, aching muscles in the lower back.
- Massages and invigorates the lower body.

Directions

1. Stand up straight with your feet at least twelve inches apart and put your hands on your hips.

2. Bending the knees slightly, stretch your right hip to the side and hold it there for fifteen seconds.

3. Extend your buttocks out in back of you, holding your shoulders steady. Hold them there for fifteen seconds.

4. Stretch your left hip to the left side and hold it there for fifteen seconds.

5. Stretch your tummy forward and hold it there for fifteen seconds.

6. Now put all these movements together in a full hip rotation. Move the hips slowly around to the right for one minute (see Figure 7.70) and around to the left for another thirty seconds.

7. Come to a standstill and take 2-3 "Rock the Baby" breaths (see page 19).

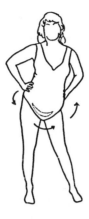

Figure 7.70 The Hip Rotator

Cautions and Comments

• You should be moving only your hips, not your shoulders. (To check, put your hands on your shoulders and see if they are moving.)

• This "belly dancing" movement is a favorite of pregnant women.

• You can do this movement in the shower each morning to make sure you have a backache-free day.

Pregnancy Triangle

Benefits

• Relieves backache while stretching and strengthening the spine.
• Tones the hip, thigh, buttocks, and leg muscles.
• Keeps at least part of your waistline intact.
• Keeps your shoulders limber.
• Stretches the pectoralis group, obliques and rectus abdominalis, the hip adductors, the hamstrings, the soleus (on side of bent knee) muscles.
• Tones and strengthens abdominals (all sections), scapular and shoulder girdle muscles on either side of the trunk, the triceps brachii, the quadraceps, the hamstrings and hip adductor muscles.

Directions

1. Separate your feet (at least 3-4 feet apart).

2. Turn your right foot on a 90° angle, and the left foot on a 45° angle facing in toward the right foot.

3. Stretch your arms out straight from your shoulders on either side, stretching the right arm as far over to the right as you can. Bend your right knee. Feel a good stretch (see Figure 7.71).

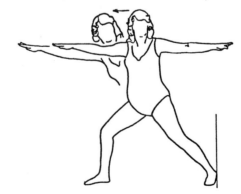

Figure 7.71 Getting Ready for the Pregnancy Triangle

4. Allow the right arm and hand to come down on your right leg. Put your left hand on your left hip (see Figure 7.72).

5. Push your hip back and feel a good stretch in the groin. Try to make the pelvic area as flat as you can.

6. Stretch the left arm straight up toward the ceiling. Your left arm should be right next to your left ear.

7. Stretch the left arm so that it is parallel to the floor on the right side, as you place your hand next to your right foot. Keep the left arm near the left ear (see Figure 7.72).

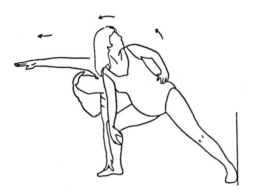

Figure 7.72   The Completed Pregnancy Triangle

8. Allow your body to come down a little bit lower on the right side. Keep the left arm steady and straight, with your fingertips together.

9. Slowly allow the left arm to come back into the air. Bend the right knee. Put your right hand on your right knee and push on your right knee until you feel yourself slowly coming up.

10. Let the left arm come down. Take a breath and let it go.

11. Now shift the left foot onto a 90° angle, and the right foot onto a 45° angle, facing toward the left. Repeat the same exercise on the other side.

Cautions and Comments

• In the later months of pregnancy, a simpler version of the Pregnancy Triangle might be necessary. Begin with your legs four feet apart. Do not bend your legs. Place your right hand on your right knee, pushing your left hip back as far as you can. Then stretch the left arm next to your left ear, stretching directly to the right side. Breathing normally, hold the stretch from thirty seconds to one minute (see Figure 7.73). Exhaling and coming up, take 2-3 "Rock the Baby" breaths (see page 19) and repeat on the other side.

• During the later months, you may want to have a chair next to you to help you get back up.

• You can maximize the stretch to your waist by stretching the top arm further forward.

• Don't let the top arm droop toward the floor; always keep it parallel to the floor and stretched.

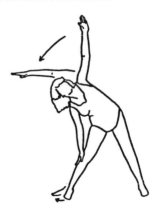

Figure 7.73   A Simpler Version of Pregnancy Triangle

Side Lunge

Benefits

- Tones, firms, and stretches the inner thighs, legs, buttocks, and arms.
- Helps to strengthen and stretch the birth canal area (pelvic floor muscles).
- Reduces tension and stiffness in the arms, neck, and back.
- Variation I: Stretches the hip adductors, the perineal muscles (pelvic floor), the hamstrings, the soleus muscle (Achilles tendon) on the bent knee. Variation II: Stretches the pectoralis muscles, the triceps brachii and the abdominal muscles.
- Variation I: Tones and strengthens the quadraceps, the hip adductors, the gastrocnemius-soleus muscles, the gluteal muscles. Variation II: Tones and strengthens the postvertebrals (erector spinae), parascapular (trapezii, rhomboideus) muscles.

Directions for Variation I

1. Standing straight, with your legs as wide open as is comfortable, lean your left foot up against a wall. Turn your right foot out 90° to the side.

2. Bending your right leg, shift your weight to your right leg and lunge over to the right side (see Figure 7.74). Keep your left leg straight, tightening your knee.

3. Hold for 5-30 seconds; breathe normally.

4. Return to starting position. Take 1-3 "Rock the Baby" breaths (see page 19). Repeat on other side.

5. Practice 2-3 stretches on each side.

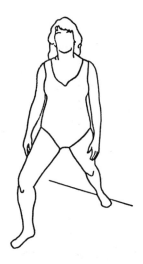

Figure 7.74   Side Lunge—Variation I

Directions for Variation II

1. Once you have assumed a lunge position as described in #1-3 above, turn at the waist toward the right side.

2. Stretch your arms out to the sides and then place your palms together above your head as you inhale.

3. Stretch the arms up as you look at your hands and breathe normally. Maximize your stretch and hold for 5-30 seconds (see Figure 7.75).

4. Exhale as you release the arms and return to starting position.

5. Take 2-3 "Rock the Baby" breaths (see page 19) and repeat on the other side.

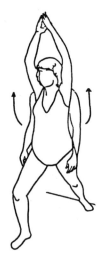

Figure 7.75 Side Lunge with Arm
Stretch—Variation II

Cautions and Comments

- Try to keep the outstretched leg straight and foot flat on the floor.
- In Variation II, move your arms behind your head to maximize the stretch to your lower back.

STANDING EXERCISES WITH A CHAIR

When you are pregnant, you may often feel the urge to really stretch the lower back and spine. Since you cannot practice any postures lying flat on your abdomen, standing exercises are a very useful substitute. Do not limit yourself to a chair for practice. Using the side of the sink during dishwashing breaks will work just as well. Also try to find other creative places to practice these stretches. (By the way, these tension-releasing movements work well at 2:00 A.M., when you just can't seem to get back to sleep.)

The Balanced Mother

Benefits

- Promotes better balance during pregnancy.
- Relieves tired legs.
- Strengthens and tones the gluteus medius, the gastrocnemius-soleus muscle groups, lumbar and thoracic postvertebrals (erector spinae), the deltoideus, the middle and lower trapezius muscles.
- Stretches the guadraceps, the ankle and footlong extensors (anterior tibialis and extensor digitorum), the iliopsoas, the pectoralis major, and the deltoideus muscles.

Directions

1. Stand up straight and tall. Shift all your weight to your left leg. Grasp a chair with your left hand and reach back to clasp your right leg with your right hand (see Figure 7.76).

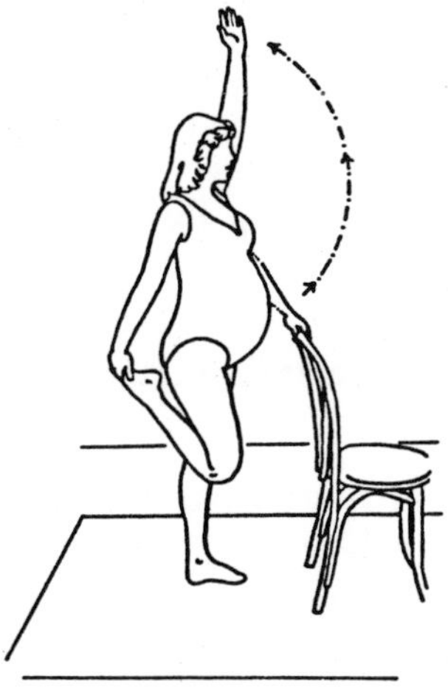

Figure 7.76   The Balanced Mother

2. Concentrate on a spot three feet in front of you. Hold onto the chair until you think you are balanced.

3. Slowly lift your hand from the chair and reach for the ceiling (see Figure 7.76).

4. Balance there for thirty seconds to one minute.

5. Slowly bring your left arm and right foot down and relax. Take two "Rock the Baby" breaths (see page 19).

6. Repeat on the other side.

Cautions and Comments

•Women with varicose veins can do this exercise, being careful not to hold the bent leg too close to the buttocks. Simply bend the leg as in Figure 7.77.

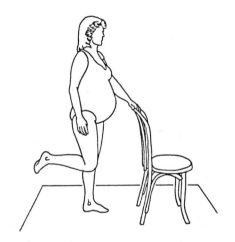

Figure 7.77   Position for Women with Varicose Veins

•Practicing this exercise will make you more limber and graceful.
•You may find that balancing is easier on one leg than on the other.

The Fruitful Tree Pose

Benefits

- Promotes better balance during pregnancy.
- Relieves tired legs.
- Stretches the hip adductors and the perineal region, the latissimus dorsi, the lower trapezius muscles.
- Tones and strengthens the quadraceps, the gastrocnemius-soleus muscle groups of the support leg and the iliopsoas muscle group of the raised leg.
- Strengthens the thoracic postvertebrals, the middle deltoideus and upper trapezius muscles.

Directions for Variation I

1. Stand up straight, twelve inches to the side of the chair, holding onto the chair with the right hand. Keep your legs close together.

2. Shifting your weight onto your left leg, slowly reach down and draw up your right leg into your groin area (see Figure 7.78).

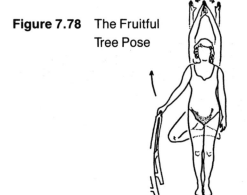

Figure 7.78 The Fruitful Tree Pose

3. Holding onto the chair, try to balance on your left leg for thirty seconds to one minute by concentrating on a spot three feet in front of you.

4. Return the right leg to the starting position and take 2-3 "Rock the Baby" breaths (see page 19). Repeat on the other side.

Directions for Variation II

1. After you have assumed the Simple Tree Pose described in Directions #1-3 above, try to get your balance and slowly move your hands up into the air, together or apart. Concentrate on a spot three feet in front of you to hold your balance.

2. Hold this pose for thirty seconds and bring the hands down slowly without losing your balance.

3. Take 2-3 "Rock the Baby" breaths (see page 19) and proceed to the other side.

Cautions and Comments

- Women with varicose veins should *not* practice this pose because it puts too much strain on the veins.
- Balancing when you are pregnant is difficult because your center of balance is constantly changing.
- This challenging pose is included in the PPF program because, when you finally master it, *it feels so good!*

Half Bow with Chair

Benefits

- Gives a stimulating stretch to the lower back, thereby releasing tension.
- Tones and tightens the thighs, hips, and buttocks.
- Helps to prevent groin spasms (round ligament spasms).
- Strengthens the shoulders and arms.
- Helps to eliminate middle-of-the-night insomnia.
- Stretches the abdominals (primarily rectus abdominalis), the iliopsoas muscle groups, the quadraceps (primarily rectus femoris), the pectoralis major, the biceps brachii.
- Tones and strengthens the hamstrings and hip adductor muscles.

Directions

1. Stand up straight, twelve inches behind a chair. Place your right hand on top of the chair.

2. Shift your weight to your right leg, keeping it straight but not locked.

3. Bend your left leg up and place your left hand on the top part of your left foot (see Figure 7.79).

4. Keep your left arm straight as you pull the left leg up and open it as wide as you can (see Figure 7.79).

5. Breathe normally as you hold this posture for 5-30 seconds.

6. Lower the left knee down and release your left foot.

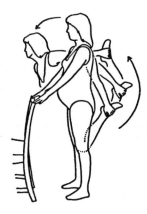

Figure 7.79   Half Bow with Chair

7. With both feet on the ground, take 2-3 "Rock the Baby" breaths (see page 19).

8. Repeat on other side.

Cautions and Comments

- Bending the arm that is on the chair will give you better balance.
- You can turn your head and look back at your raised foot for an added stretch to the neck area.
- This is a tension-releasing posture which can be used as a quick energizer.
- This can easily be done near your sink if your lower back begins to ache as you do the dishes.
- You can do this stretch with your leg outstretched and both hands on top of the chair. But you should hold the leg lift for only 5-30 seconds on each side.

The Scale

Benefits

- Strengthens your legs.
- Promotes a sense of balance all through pregnancy.
- Variation I: Tones the quadraceps, the gastrocnemius-soleus muscle complex, adductors (gluteus medius), hamstrings, gluteus maximus, the rectus and oblique abdominals, lower lumbar muscle group, the postvertebrals (erector spinae).
- Variation II: Strengthens the gluteus maximus, the hamstrings and the lumbar postvertebrals (erector spinae).

Directions for Variation I

1. Stand up straight and tall. Holding onto a chair, shift your weight onto your left foot.

2. Bend your right leg back. Concentrate on a spot three feet in front of you and try to balance (see Figure 7.80).

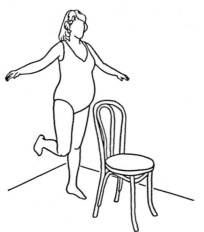

Figure 7.80 The Scale—Variation I

3. Spreading your arms to the side to keep your balance, balance in this position for fifteen seconds to one minute.

4. Bring the right leg down. Take 1-2 "Rock the Baby" breaths (see page 19) and repeat the entire exercise on the other side.

Directions for Variation II

1. Proceed through Directions #1-2 in Variation I, but continue to hold onto the chair as you raise the right leg higher in the air behind you. Lean toward the chair as you stretch your right arm straight out from the right shoulder (see Figure 7.81).

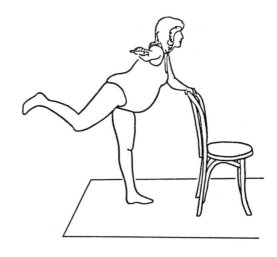

Figure 7.81 The Scale—Variation II

2. Balance while concentrating on a spot three feet in front of you. Breathe normally.

3. Hold the balance for thirty seconds to one minute.

4. Return to the starting position and take 1-2 "Rock the Baby" breaths (see page 19).

5. Repeat on the other side.

Cautions and Comments

- You will learn that it is easier to balance on one leg than on the other. Eventually you will learn to balance equally well.
- This Scale Exercise is more fun than the scale at the doctor's or midwife's office!

POSES IN A FLAT BACK POSITION

During the later months of pregnancy, you may find that lying supine on your back with the full weight of the uterus and baby pressing down on your circulatory system is very uncomfortable. Some women experience numbness in their legs if they are forced to remain still in this position for extended periods of time. Therefore, flat back resting positions are to be *avoided* during pregnancy because they can deprive your baby of oxygen. The following exercises can be safely practiced *only* during the early part of your pregnancy, but they should never be done consecutively. Immediately go into a side-lying position for breathing upon completion of each exercise. You can easily intersperse these postures with side-lying or sitting exercises. If you feel *any* discomfort within the latter half of your pregnancy, *immediately* discontinue these exercises.

Pendulum Legs

Benefits

- Massage and release tension from the lower back.
- Relieve lower backache.
- Help to tone the thighs, waist, and buttocks.
- Bring relaxation to the entire body.
- Stretch erector spinae, the gluteals, the tensor fascia latae and iliotibial tract, the oblique abdominalis, the pectoralis major, the neck rotators.
- Tone and strengthen paraspinal erector spinae muscles at all levels.

Directions

1. Lying on your back, stretch your arms straight out from your shoulders.

2. Bend both legs at the knees and put your legs together and your feet flat on the floor as close to your body as is comfortable.

3. Begin moving your knees from side to side, like a pendulum (see Figure 7.82).

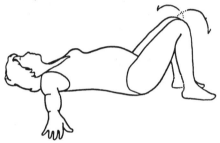

Figure 7.82 Pendulum Legs

4. Let the knees eventually fall to one side for 5-10 seconds. Repeat on other side.

5. Keep moving the knees in a pendulum motion from side to side until your lower back begins to feel warm and relaxed.

6. Shift into a side-lying position and take 2-3 "Rock the Baby" breaths (see page 19).

Cautions and Comments

- Do this exercise *only* if it feels good.
- Be sure to practice only on a well-padded mat. An extra pillow placed beneath your lower back will be helpful.
- You do not have to keep your feet on the ground as you move your knees from side to side.
- Keep your eyes closed and concentrate on the area of your back which is being massaged.
- Most pregnant women love this exercise.

Universal Pose

Benefits

- Loosens, relaxes, and tones the lower back, which can often ache during pregnancy.
- Strengthens the spine while keeping it supple.
- Tones the legs, thighs, and buttocks.

- Relieves lower backache.
- Stretches the lower lumbar postvertebrals (erector spinae), the multifidus and iliolumbar fascia, the oblique abdominalis, the pectoralis major.

Directions

1. Lying on your back, bend your left leg and place your left foot next to your inside right knee (see Figure 7.83).

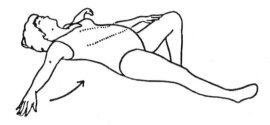

Figure 7.83 Getting Ready for the Universal Pose

2. Shift your left arm so that it extends straight out from your left shoulder.

3. Place your right hand on your left knee as you roll the left knee toward the mat on the right side. Your left hip will roll into the air.

4. Turn your head and look in the opposite direction of your knee (see Figure 7.84). Try to keep your arms and shoulders as close to the mat as is comfortable.

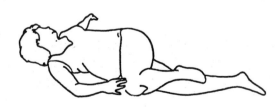

Figure 7.84 The Completed Universal Pose

5. Hold this posture for 5-30 seconds as you consciously relax your shoulders, hips, and legs. Breathe normally throughout.

6. Return to a starting position.

7. Take 2-3 "Rock the Baby" breaths (see page 19) and repeat movements on the other side. Repeat this posture twice.

Cautions and Comments

- You may hear the bones in your back crack as you practice this exercise. Do not be alarmed. You are merely breaking up calcium deposits, as well as releasing bodily tension and tiredness.
- You may find that bending the bottom leg a bit more will increase your enjoyment of this exercise.
- If the top leg does not want to go down to the mat, you can rest it on a pillow (see Figure 7.85) for a comforting stretch.

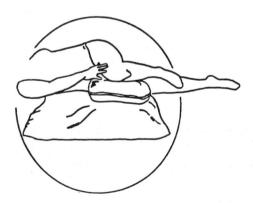

Figure 7.85 Pillows and the Universal Pose

EXERCISES IN A SITTING POSITION

The bigger you grow, the more difficult it becomes to sit in any one position for a long period of time. A variety of sitting positions have already been described and illustrated in the Salute to the Child exercise. In addition, there are a number of other positions which can be most helpful when you cannot seem to find a comfortable way to sit. If you become familiar with and use these sitting positions from the early months of your pregnancy, you should experience more comfort as you grow. Sitting cross-legged is excellent for strengthening your thigh and perineal muscles in preparation for childbirth. However, if you have varicose veins, cross-legged sitting is *not* advised. Use the "Zen Sitting Position" (p. 126) and the "Butterfly" (p. 99) instead. Try to use the following suggestions to increase your physical comfort while sitting during pregnancy.

- When sitting in a chair, bend one leg at the knee and place the foot of the bent leg on the chair next to the other thigh; after a while, shift legs so the other leg is bent.
- If you are sitting for long periods of time, put your legs up on another chair or an ottoman.
- Change sitting positions often.
- Sit cross-legged on the floor as often as possible during your leisure time. Try it on the sofa. If you have varicose veins, use the Zen Sitting Position.
- Be sure your back is supported when you are sitting for long periods of time.

When you are unable to sit in yoga sitting positions and must use conventional chairs, you should pay even more attention to your sitting posture. As the center of your body balloons out, there is a tendency for your head to drop forward and for you to develop the "pregnancy slouch." This dreaded postural condition can only lead to one thing: *backache!* Compare Figures 7.86 and 7.87.

When you are not sitting on a chair or sofa, you may want to use a Seiza bench. This Japanese bench was invented to enable people to sit comfortably for long periods of meditation. During the last trimester, when comfort is just a fading memory, this bench can become your favorite sitting place.

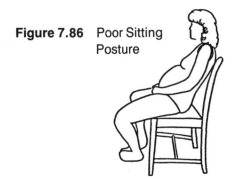

Figure 7.86 Poor Sitting Posture

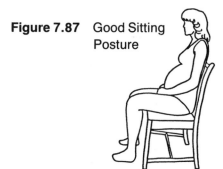

Figure 7.87 Good Sitting Posture

Alternate Leg Stretch to the Side

Benefits

- •Strengthens and firms the abdomen and legs.
- •Relieves and reduces tension in the back, legs, and buttocks.
- •The abdominal organs are massaged and stimulated into action for better digestion and elimination.
- •Energizes the body by making the spine strong and flexible.
- •Stretches the hip adductors, the hamstrings, the gastroc-soleus muscle complex, and the latissimus dorsi.
- •Tones and strengthens the oblique abdominalis, the lower back postvertebrals (erector spinae) muscles, the quadraceps.

Directions

1. Sit on your mat with a straight back in the open "V" leg position. Take 1-2 "Rock the Baby" breaths (see page 19).

2. Clasp your hands and inhale while bringing your hands up above your head (see Figure 7.88).

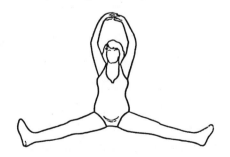

Figure 7.88   Preparation for Alternate Leg Stretch to the Side

3. Breathing normally and keeping your head between your upper arms, stretch as far down toward the extended leg as is comfortable. Do not hold your breath or bounce. Hold for 5-30 seconds (see Figure 7.89).

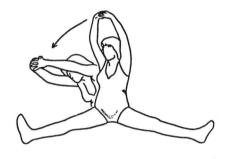

Figure 7.89   Completed Alternate Leg Stretch to the Side

4. Stretch back up into an upright position. Exhale as you lower your hands back down to your knees.

5. Take 2-3 "Rock the Baby" breaths (see page 19) and then repeat movements on the other side.

Cautions and Comments

- •During the early months of your pregnancy, you may find it quite easy to lower your head quite close to your knee. But as the baby grows, you may find it uncomfortable to stretch down quite so far. You can hold a towel looped around your foot for increased stretch to the gastroc-soleus (calf) muscles.

- This exercise is highly beneficial for eliminating middle and lower back pain.
- If your knee hurts too much, you can bend the knee that isn't in the groin area. This should relieve the pain.
- This exercise can also be practiced with the legs in an open "V" position, with one hand extended and touching the toes or calf of the same leg, and the other hand stretched above and parallel to it (see Figure 7.90).

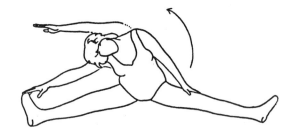

Figure 7.90   Alternate Leg Stretch in an Open "V" Position

Cow Head Pose

Benefits

- Helps to improve rounded shoulders and poor posture.
- Helps to counterbalance the extra weight of your breasts.
- Strengthens and firms your upper arms.
- Releases tension in the shoulders while exercising the muscles near your shoulder blades and in the upper back.
- Stretches the triceps brachii, the lower trapezius, the pectoralis major, the posterior deltoideus, the latissimus dorsi, the oblique abdominalis, the anterior and middle deltoideus, the rotator cuff muscles, the upper trapezius.
- Tones and strengthens all portions of the deltoideus and trapezius muscle groups, the triceps brachii, the pectoralis major, the rotator cuff muscles.

Directions

1. Sit straight in any comfortable position.

2. Bend your left arm and bring it behind your back, with your palm facing out. Try to move it as far up your back as you can.

3. Bring your right arm straight up and bend it, trying to bring it to the center of your back.

4. Try to bring your hands as close together as you can and eventually interlock the hands (see Figure 7.91).

5. Keep the top elbow straight up in the air, so that it resembles a cow's horn.

6. Hold for 5-30 seconds, or as long as is comfortable. Gently pull upward with the right hand, then downward with the left hand. Breathe normally throughout.

7. Separate the hands and repeat on the other side. Repeat the entire exercise twice.

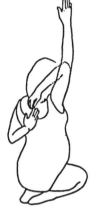

Figure 7.91 The Cow Head Pose

Cautions and Comments

•Do not be dismayed if you cannot clasp your hands. Simply hold a small towel or handkerchief in the top hand, clasp it with the bottom hand, and stretch (see Figure 7.92). Eventually, the hands will clasp.

•If you are right-handed, you will probably find that the left side is very difficult to clasp. The opposite is true for left-handed people.

•This is an excellent exercise for pregnant women who are working at a desk. It will reduce accumulated tension in the shoulders.

•Remember to keep your back straight.

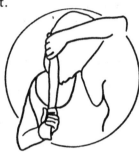

Figure 7.92 Using a Towel in the Cow Head Pose

Cross-Legged Sitting Positions

Benefits

•Improve circulation in your legs.
•Strengthen the muscles of the thighs, legs, and spine.
•Increase flexibility of the ankles, knees, and hip joints.
•Improve your posture.
•Stretch the hip adductors, the hip internal rotators, quadraceps.
•Strengthen the erector spinae muscles (postvertebrals) of the entire spine, the abdominalis muscles.

Directions for Simple Cross-Legged Sitting

1. Sit with your knees bent out to the side, ankles crossed in a simple cross-legged position. Place your hands on your knees (see Figure 7.93).

2. Check to see that your spine is straight. If your back is aching, use a wall for support.

3. Remain in this position for as long as is comfortable.

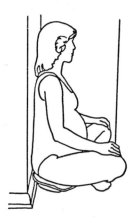

Figure 7.93 Simple Cross-Legged Sitting Position

Directions for Half Lotus Position

1. Sit up tall, with both legs stretching forward.

2. Bend the left leg and place the left heel as close to the right thigh and the birth canal as possible.

3. Take the right foot in both hands and place it on your left thigh so that the right foot is resting on the crevice created between your left thigh and calf.

4. Place your hands on your knees and practice your breathing, watch television, read, etc.

5. Hold each side for thirty seconds to five minutes, then change to the other side.

6. When finishing this pose, stretch your legs forward and vibrate your knees.

Cautions and Comments

- If you have varicose veins, all cross-legged sitting positions should be discontinued. Use a Seiza bench, the Zen Sitting Position, or sit in a chair with your feet up.
- If you are comfortable using a cross-legged sitting position, try it on a wide chair while eating dinner.
- Sitting cross-legged will help to strengthen your spine and take some pressure off your lower back.
- Use a cushion under your buttocks if the floor is too hard.

Elbow Circles

Benefits

- Loosen, relax, and release tension from the shoulders and lower neck areas.
- Help to prevent headaches.
- Stretch the upper thoracic spine postvertebrals, the pectoralis major, the triceps brachii muscles.
- Tone and strengthen the biceps bra-

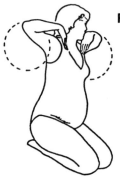

Figure 7.94 Elbow Circles

chii, the middle deltoideus, the upper trapezius, the rotator cuff muscles.

Directions

1. Bend your arms and place the palms of your hands on your shoulders, with your fingers facing in toward your neck.

2. Begin to make circles with your elbows (see Figure 7.94).

3. Make five very large circles forward. Reverse and make five circles backwards.

4. Bring your hands back into your lap and take 1-2 "Rock the Baby" breaths (see page 19).

Cautions and Comments

- This posture is highly recommended for women who work at desks or at any job which requires forward bending. Use it often during your work day.
- You can try an interesting variation by pushing the elbows as far behind you as you can, keeping your hands on your shoulders. Hold for a count of five and then move the elbows in front of you. Hold again for a count of five as you touch your elbows together. Release and breathe.
- You may hear cracking in the shoulder area as you practice this pose. This is a sign of tightness, which you are breaking up.

The Inclined Plane with Baby

Benefits

- Strengthens the arms, shoulders, and back.
- Is a very powerful and energizing posture.
- Stretches the biceps brachii, the anterior deltoideus, the pectoralis major, the anterior chest wall, the anterior neck muscles (sternocleido-mastoideus), scaleni muscle group, iliopsoas muscles.
- Tones and strengthens the gluteus maximus, the hamstrings, all levels of the postvertebral (erector spinae) muscles of the spine, the rhomboideus muscle group, the middle trapezius, the latissimus dorsi.

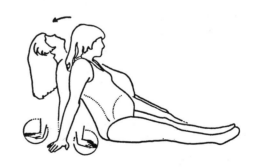

Figure 7.95 The Inclined Plane with Baby

Directions

1. Sitting upright on your mat, feet together, place your arms shoulder distance apart (either facing out to the side, in back of you, or in front of you—whatever is most comfortable for you). See Figure 7.95.

2. Take a deep breath. On the exhalation, lift your entire body up in the air as you bend your head back a little. Your spine should look like an inclined plane.

3. Keep breathing normally for thirty seconds and carefully ease yourself down.

4. Shake your hands out and take 2-3 "Rock the Baby" breaths (see page 19).

5. Repeat this exercise 2-3 more times.

Cautions and Comments

- When you first try this exercise, you may only be able to do it for fifteen seconds. With practice you will be able to hold it longer.
- Toward the end of your pregnancy, your bodily weight may prevent you from practicing this posture at all.
- If you tend to get dizzy, keep your head facing forward in Direction #2 above.

Moving the Balloon

Benefits

- Strengthens the arm and shoulder muscles.
- Tones the thigh and calf muscles.
- Develops your concentration skills.
- Stretches the hip adductors, the perineal muscles (pelvic floor), the hamstrings, the oblique abdominalis, the sternal portion of the pectoralis major, the anterior neck muscles.
- Tones and strengthens the postvertebral (erector spinae) muscles at all levels of the spine, the middle and lower trapezii, the serratus anterior, the deltoideus (anterior portion), the pectoralis major, the rotator cuff muscle group, the biceps and triceps brachii muscle groups.

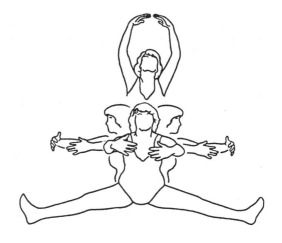

Figure 7.96   Moving the Balloon

Directions

1. Sitting up straight in a "V" sitting position with the legs apart, raise your hands in front of you as if you're holding a large balloon.

2. Slowly bring the balloon out in front of you (see Figure 7.96).

3. Now stretch the balloon as far to one side as is comfortable. Hold it there, breathing normally for thirty seconds.

4. Stretch the other side, moving slowly and gracefully, and hold it there for thirty seconds.

5. Coming back to center, finally stretch the balloon up above your head and slowly lower it to the ground very carefully.

6. Take 2-3 "Rock the Baby" breaths (see page 19) and relax.

Cautions and Comments

•This exercise can really tone your arms and make them strong in a very short time. You'd be surprised at how much baby equipment weighs!
•In the later months, you may experience numbness in your arms when you lift them above your head. Keep on practicing the right and left movements.
•Moving slowly and really concentrating on what you are doing will give you a better stretch.
•Try it a second time, stretching even further.

Pose of the Moon

Benefits

•Improves flexibility in the legs and knees.
•Releases tension in the shoulders and arms.
•Gently stretches and strengthens the spine and back muscles.
•Is a quick energizer.
•Stretches all portions of the pectoralis major and anterior chest wall, the lower and middle trapezius, the latissimus dorsi, the lower lumbar spine postvertebrals (erector spinae), the gluteus maximus, the quadraceps, the hip adductors and the perineal muscles (pelvic floor).

•Tones and strengthens the cervical and thoracic postvertebrals (erector spinae), the rhomboideus muscle group, and the upper trapezius.

Directions

1. Sit in the Zen Sitting Position by bending both legs and sitting on your heels. Separate your knees so they are 6-8 inches apart.

2. Sit up straight, raising both arms. Stretch as high above your head as possible.

3. Hold the stretch as you move your arms down to the floor in front of you. Place your forehead on the mat (see Figure 7.97).

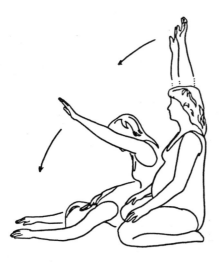

Figure 7.97   The Three Phases of Pose of the Moon

4. Stretch your arms and fingers as far in front of you as is comfortable. Breathe normally as you hold for 10-60 seconds.

5. Stretch the arms back up into the air and then float them down to your sides as you exhale.

6. Repeat twice.

Cautions and Comments

•As the pregnancy progresses, you may want to have a pillow on the floor for your head.

•When the uterus is expanded to its highest height, usually during the eighth and ninth months, you may find this exercise uncomfortable.

•This posture can easily be done at your desk if you work in an office. It is very effective as an energizer and tension-releaser.

Sitting on a Seiza Bench

Benefits

•Will force your spine into correct alignment, which will cause your back to feel wonderful.

•Ideal for women with varicose veins.

•Releases tension from the neck and shoulders.

•Increases flexibility in your knees and legs.

•Enables you to find a comfortable position for meditation periods.

•Stretches the quadraceps, the long toe extensors (dorsiflexors).

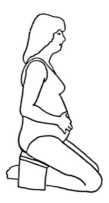

Figure 7.98   Sitting on a Seiza Bench

Directions

1. Resting on your knees, place both feet together. Place the Seiza bench over your lower legs and feet.

2. Lower your bottom onto the bench and sit up straight (see Figure 7.98).

3. Use this position for meditation or to watch television, etc.

Cautions and Comments

• You can put a cushion on the top of the bench for more comfort.

• You can read in this position using a coffee table for a book rest.

• A Seiza bench is available through PPF. See the Appendix.

EXERCISES FOR THE PELVIC FLOOR OR BIRTH CANAL MUSCLES

Prior to pregnancy, the muscles of the pelvic floor are used for eliminative and sexual purposes. With the advent of the growing uterus and impending birth, these muscles become much more significant. You may have gone through your life up until now not really being aware that you have a layer of muscles which form a sling or support system across the bottom of your pelvis. The easiest way to familiarize yourself with these muscles is to do the Elevator.

The Elevator

Benefits

• Strengthens the muscles that will be used during childbirth.
• Exercises all the inner muscles of the pelvic floor.
• Helps to keep the sexual area alive and responsive.
• Strengthens the pelvic floor (bulbospongiosus, transverse perinei superficialis and profundus, ischiocavernosus)

Directions

1. In any comfortable position, focus your awareness on your vaginal or birth canal area muscles. Take one "Rock the Baby" breath (see page 19) and exhale.

2. Imagine that your pelvic floor muscles are an elevator that is slowly moving up from the first to the sixth floor. Slowly begin to pull your muscles up

toward your spine. You may feel a slight tightening in the lowest part of the abdomen.

3. Really concentrate and feel the muscles on the first floor, second floor, etc. Hold the elevator at the sixth floor for 5-10 seconds and then slowly lower it.

4. Control the elevator's descent to the first floor and then lower it to the basement by pushing down.

5. Repeat this trip 2-3 times, then relax as you take 2-3 "Rock the Baby" breaths (see page 19).

Cautions and Comments

- As your muscle tone increases, it will become much easier to hold the elevator at the top floor.
- After you deliver the elevator to the basement, relax all the muscles of the pelvic floor completely. You will have to be able to relax this area at will during delivery to facilitate the birth of your child.

In addition to the Elevator, see Baby Breath (page 23), the Anal Lock (page 88), and the Pelvic Exercises (page 89).

MAKING LOVE DURING PREGNANCY

The preceding exercises will focus your attention on, as well as tone and strengthen, your sexual muscles. They may also heighten your sexual desires during pregnancy. Sharing feelings about your sexuality with your mate, either verbally or via a letter, is very important for your well-being. Women commonly experience a decrease in sexual desire during the first trimester, increased interest and pleasure during the second trimester, and a decrease (due to size) during the third trimester. Keeping your husband informed of your changing desires and reactions can eliminate many problems and frustrations. Ask your mate about the desirability of your pregnant body. This exchange of ideas and opinions can have a very positive effect on your sex life while you are pregnant. New ideas and reactions will cross your minds. Many men have underlying fears of hurting the baby while making love. Many women feel the need for more closeness via hugging or massage rather than intercourse. Each couple's reactions are uniquely their own and should be explored for a more positive pregnancy experience. Reading and discussing the book, *Making Love During Pregnancy*, by Elisabeth Bing and Libby Colman (Bantam Books, 1977) can help them explore new horizons. This honest and open book contains beautiful illustrations and direct quotes from many couples concerning their sexual experiences.

You may wonder about yoga's connection with sexual activity, since many people equate strict yoga practice with celibacy. The aspect of yoga which has been developed within this book is designed especially for people in the mainstream of life, rather than those who have limited their activities. The goal of yoga practice is physical, mental, and spiritual development, and sexual relations can play a very vital part in this development.

Since pregnancy affords you freedom from birth control techniques, there can be more spontaneity in your sexual pursuits. The challenge of an ever-enlarging female body can lead to more creative lovemaking. The combination of these two factors can add new dimensions to the sexual aspect of your lives. If you have been practicing your exercises on a regular basis, you will find that you have become more flexible, and thereby capable, of holding positions for longer periods of time. Another positive aspect of pregnancy is heightened sensitivity.

The same inner energy which is responsible for your emotional ups and downs can be used quite pleasurably during lovemaking. This inner energy often increases your physical bodily responses, thereby enabling you to reach and feel deeper sexual pleasure. These responses can be used even if you are not making love. A mutual massage (see Chapter 11) can be extremely enjoyable and satisfying for both partners, if lovemaking is not feasible or desired. It is just another way of being close and giving pleasure to one another.

Pregnancy may be the first time a couple explores other ways of pleasuring each other. Developing new techniques during the middle pregnancy months may prove quite helpful during the time just before and right after your baby is born. Many women have reported feelings of pride or increased femininity upon learning to bring their mates to orgasm in a new way. Other women were relieved to know that a heightened sexual drive could be relieved by masturbation without any ill effects on the baby. Many couples discover mutual masturbation during the waiting months. These preparatory months are definitely the right time to explore and deepen your physical bodily experiences.

An opportune time to find out the strength of your birth canal (pelvic floor) muscles is during lovemaking. Simply contract your pelvic floor muscles and ask your mate about the tightness of the contraction. One husband used to suggest practicing the pelvic exercises every time he wanted to make love. His wife reported that he thought this gave the lovemaking a very noble and worthwhile purpose!

Another yogic technique which may increase or prolong your sexual pleasure is simultaneous breathing after both partners have reached orgasm. This breathing doesn't have to be deep—just mutual. Try to breathe in unison as you hold the embrace. Concentrate on the physical union that you are experiencing.

A variety of new physical positions is open to you at this time as well. As the abdomen grows larger, it may be advisable for the woman to be on top. You may find the use of a chair with an ottoman next to it quite helpful. Your husband can lie on the chair and ottoman with you above him, with your feet on the floor and hands on the ottoman. In this position, you can guide the depth of penetration as well as the rhythm of movement. This position can be adapted for the corner of the bed, again with the woman's feet on the floor (if the woman is not too tall). Other couples have indicated that rear entry positions, with the woman either lying down or standing, are helpful as well. The key word at this time is *experiment*. Try out a variety of positions and find the ones you like best.

Many women report that having followed the advice to experiment, they find themselves spending a great deal of time laughing at some of the results. Laughter and joking can add the light touch that is needed, especially during the last weeks of pregnancy. Some of your experiments may end with making jokes rather than making love, while others may be very satisfying. By keeping this area of your life as positive and light-hearted as possible, you will strengthen your marriage and come to realize new facets of the love you share.

STRETCHING AND RELAXING ON THE JOB

You may have seen some exercises in this book that you would like to practice *if* you had the time. Now that working throughout the pregnant months has become more acceptable, increasing numbers of women find themselves doing so. It is extremely difficult to fit a daily PPF practice session into a schedule that begins early in the morning and ends late in the evening. You may think about practicing and then feel very guilty because you have not gotten around to doing it. Those kinds of thoughts defeat the whole purpose of practicing. With this situation in mind, I have compiled a list of exercises that can be integrated into your working day. By including these movements during your working hours, or on your lunch breaks, you will have more energy and feel better by the end of the day. If you do get positive results, you will be much more inclined to practice the pregnancy exercises on the weekends.

Breathing Exercises

- "Rock the Baby" Breath (page 19)
- Smooth Breath (page 25)
- Sighing Breath (page 25)
- Energizing Single Nostril Breath (page 24)

STRETCHING ON THE JOB

It's a good idea to talk with your co-workers about your interest in learning the PPF program while you are pregnant. Tell them how learning to relax using the program can help to shorten your laboring time. I don't mean to develop a vocal group of PPF admirers, but rather to eliminate the strange looks you may receive if a co-worker walks in while you are practicing one of the following exercises.

A WORD OF CAUTION: There is some evidence that working at a computer terminal may cause birth defects in your child because of the radiation that is given off by the computer. More studies dealing with this matter are currently in progress. If your job requires computer work and you are worried about the possible danger to your child, perhaps you should consider switching jobs or at least being given another task. The health of your growing baby depends a lot on your surrounding environment.

Keep the following in mind: If you sit a great deal at work, put your feet up on a foot stool or a chair to prevent heavy, tired legs. Be sure to take a 1-2 minute walk around the office every hour to keep your body invigorated and improve your circulation. Also keep nutritious snacks handy to combat "during-the-day munchies."

Neck, Shoulder and Arm Stretches

- Neck Smiles (page 72)
- Cow Head Pose (page 120)
- Chest Expansion (page 90)
- Elbow Circles (page 122)
- Pose of the Moon (page 125)

Back Stretches

- Sitting Spinal Twist: Sitting at your desk or in a chair that has a steady back, turn around and place both hands on the top of the chair. Keep your feet and legs facing forward. Look over your back shoulder and relax those muscles that are not being used. Hold for 5-30 seconds. Return to center, take one or two "Rock the Baby" breaths (see page 19), and relax. Repeat on the other side. This exercise strengthens the spine while it simultaneously eliminates tiredness. It also helps to improve your posture.

Foot and Calf Stretches

- Foot Circles: Sitting at your desk or in a chair, slowly begin to rotate your feet at the ankle. Make five circles in one direction. Change directions and do another five circles. Then consciously relax the feet: Start with the toes and slowly work your way up the foot until your feet feel tingly and light. Foot circles increase circulation to the ankles and feet. They also help eliminate tired, aching feet.
- Foot Rolls: Stand twelve inches behind your chair. Place your hands on the back of the chair. Go up on your toes. Hold for five seconds. Shift onto the outsides of your feet. Hold for five seconds. Shift onto the heels of your feet (lift rest of foot up) and hold for five seconds; shift onto the insides of the feet (go knock-kneed) and hold for five seconds. Repeat twice. Your feet should feel cooler and lighter. This increases circulation to the feet and legs, helps to eliminate tired and swollen legs and feet, and is an energizing posture.
- Calf Stretches: Sitting at your desk or in a chair, straighten your legs and raise them about 12-15 inches off the ground. Push your heels forward and point your toes toward your knees. Hold for 20-60 seconds and release. Repeat twice. Take one or two "Rock the Baby" breaths (see page 19) between stretches, then return to work. These stretches help prevent cramping in the calf area, which is so prevalent in pregnancy. They also help to keep the legs in good tone.

WEIGHT TRAINING FOR PREGNANCY

Weight training can be quite helpful during pregnancy, for it can help to strengthen your arms, upper back and shoulders. These areas will be used extensively (especially during the first few weeks after childbirth) and should be built up prior to your baby's arrival. Should your baby be born via Cesarean section, you'll need strong arm and shoulder muscles to enable you to get into a sitting position without causing additional abdominal pain. Preparation during pregnancy for the aftermath of birth will make your recuperation period much shorter.

Benefits of Weight Training

Weight training can be a useful and vital part of your PPF exercise program. Many women do not realize the importance of upper body strength, which will come in handy before, during, and after pregnancy. Upper body strengthening not only tones and firms the arms; when practiced properly, it strengthens your shoulders, neck, chest and back while helping to maintain and develop good posture. When you use weights for upper body conditioning, your heart also benefits, for the weight training exercises included in this chapter increase stroke volume (or the amount of blood being pumped in the heart). These weight training exercises can serve as a controlled, modified, cardiovascular workout for the pregnant woman. When light weights are used properly, the quality of the workout becomes far more important than the quantity of exercises you do.

Rules for Weight Training

1. *Consult your doctor or midwife* before beginning the PPF Weight Training Program.
2. *Do not hold your breath*—breathe out during exertion and inhale when release takes place.
3. Drink at least 8 ounces of additional water daily to prevent dehydration during weight training.
4. Wear loose, comfortable clothing.
5. *Do not* use weights if you have high blood pressure or low blood sugar.
6. *Do not* exceed two pounds of weights per arm.
7. If you have neck or lower back problems, use extra caution when beginning a weight training program. It is wise to see how your body reacts to weight training. If you experience any *pain*, stop immediately.
8. Keep in mind that proper alignment is essential for safety and proper results.

9.   Stop immediately if you experience dizziness, nausea, heart palpitations, or severe and/or unusual pain.

10.   *Do not* practice weight training on a full stomach.

11.   Be sure to take 1-2 "Rock the Baby" breaths (see page 19) between each exercise.

Rules for Proper Body Alignment

1.   *Always* stand with your feet shoulder-width apart, toes slightly turned out. *Do not overextend*.

2.   *Always* stand with your back straight and pelvic area tilted forward. Your weight should be felt in the front thigh, *not* on the knees (see Figure 7.2).

3.   *Always* turn or tilt your pelvic area slightly so that you are not swayed or arched. A swayed or arched position can cause hyperextension in the back and knees. Your body should be balanced.

4.   Your shoulders should *not* be hunched and tense; they should be relaxed and even.

5.   Your neck and head should be level—not bent forward.

Recommended Weights to Use

Spenco Bio Soft Aerobic Wrist Weights, one pound each, are flexible, easy to use, and completely washable. They do not cause undue stress on your muscles, ligaments, and tendons. These weights feel properly balanced, and do not slip on your arm. The Heavy Hands (the ones used in the line drawings in this chapter) are also comfortable and easy to use. Weights can be purchased at most running shops and fitness clubs.

How Many Should I Do?

The amount of repetitions you do depends on your level of fitness. When beginning a weight training program, you should do no more than 6-8 repetitions at a time. Slowly build up the number of repetitions that you do. When you can do eight repetitions easily, you can do two sets of eight instead of one. You do not need to do more than twenty repetitions. You should always remain in control, doing slow, steady, and fluid repetitions (no jerky movements!).

Music To Train By

Mellow pop, jazz, or modified disco with no more than 120 beats per minute work well with weight training. Be creative with your music—let it suit your mood. Try ethnic, country, or even modified classical music.

   Just remember: body alignment, breathing, and concentration!

Tips For Weight Training

1. Weight training should be done in slow, methodic, steady, fluid movements. *Avoid short, jerky movements.*

2. Quality, not quantity, is important. A weight workout develops muscle strength. Do not practice fast, jerky movements that rely only on momentum.

3. Use a full range of motion during your exercises. However, modify your practice if unusual pain develops.

4. *Be sure to take 1-2 ''Rock the Baby'' breaths (see page 19) between each exercise!*

5. If you are uncomfortable standing for weight training practice, sit in a straight-backed chair and proceed with these exercises.

Some Enjoyable Weight Training Exercises

Bicep Curl

Benefits

- Strengthens and tones the biceps brachii, the brachialis, the brachiorachialis, the forearm and wrist flexors.
- Increases upper body strength.

Directions

1. Stand with your feet shoulder-distance apart, knees soft, pelvic area tilted, back straight, shoulders pushed down and relaxed, arms in front.

2. Curl the weights toward your body, being careful not to lift your elbows for a 4-8 count. You should exhale coming up and inhale coming down (see Figure 7.99).

3. Repeat to a count of eight.

Cautions and Comments

- Exhaling through an open mouth makes these weight training exercises easier to do.
- You should do no more than sixteen repetitions, preferably two sets of eight repetitions each.
- Don't hold your breath.
- Don't arch or sway your back, making sure your pelvis is tilted.
- Stop if you feel any unusual pain, nausea or dizziness.

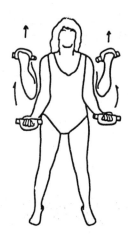

Figure 7.99 Bicep Curl

Bicep Raises

Benefits

- Strengthen and tone the biceps brachii, the brachialis and the forearm/wrist flexors, the coraco brachialis, the anterior middle deltoideus, the upper trapezius muscles.
- A good exercise for overall upper body conditioning.

Directions

1. Maintain proper body alignment (see Bicep Curl).

2. Extend arms at your sides clasping the weights. Inhale and bring the weights up to your shoulder. Exhale, bringing the weights above your head. Inhale, bringing the weights down to your shoulders and exhale bringing the weights to original position (see Figure 7.100).

3. Repeat 4-8 times. Breathe and rest.

Cautions and Comments

- Coordinate this routine with slow music to make sure that you are breathing correctly.

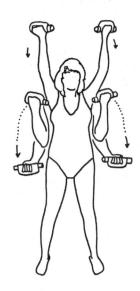

Figure 7.100 Bicep Raiser

- Do not sway your back—maintain pelvic tilt.
- Do not lock your elbows or hunch your shoulders, making sure that you keep your movements fluid.
- Stop if you feel dizzy or lightheaded. Keep breathing deeply and slowly.

Pectoral Expander and Strengthener

Benefits

- Increases chest expansion.
- Conditions the pectoral muscles which support the breasts.
- Strengthens and stretches the pectoralis major and minor, the biceps brachii, the anterior deltoideus, the coraco brachialis, the middle and lower trapezius muscles, the rhomboideus muscle group, the serratus anterior and the latissimus dorsi muscles.

Directions

1. Maintain proper body alignment (see Bicep Curl).

2. Extend your arms in front of you and bend your elbows (see Figure 7.101).

3. Using slight resistance, bring your arms together in the front, making sure not to hunch your shoulders. Your arms will touch. Exhale.

4. Bring your arms to the side as you inhale.

5. Practice 4-8 repetitions and then rest and breathe.

Cautions and Comments

- Do not sway back as you maintain the pelvic tilt.

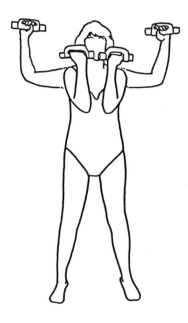

Figure 7.101   Pectoral Expander

- Do not exceed sixteen repetitions.
- Shoulders must remain relaxed, not hunched up.
- Do not hold your breath. Instead, maintain steady breathing.

Side Stretchers

Benefits

- Help condition your external and internal oblique abdominalis muscles.
- Strengthen and tone the arms and shoulders.
- Make it easier to regain your pre-pregnancy shape after your baby is born.

Directions

1. Maintain proper body alignment (see Bicep Curl).

2. Inhale as you stretch your right hand toward the outside of your right knee, while simultaneously bringing your left hand underneath your left armpit (see Figure 7.102).

3. Exhale as you practice the same movement on the other side.

4. Practice 4-8 repetitions and then rest and breathe.

Cautions and Comments

- Do not exceed sixteen repetitions.
- Bend over to your side, rather than to the front.

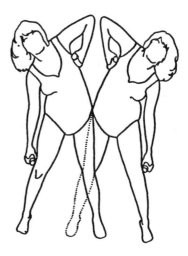

Figure 7.102   Side Stretchers

- Practice this routine with slow music to coordinate your breathing with the music.
- Breathe out through your mouth in order to make this routine easier.
- Some pregnant women become dizzy while practicing this routine. Stop immediately if you do.

Tricep Extension

Benefits

- Strengthens and tones the back of your arm.
- Exercises the opposing muscle.
- Strengthens the triceps brachii, the middle deltoideus, the upper trapezius muscles.
- Keeps upper body flexible.

Directions

1. Maintain proper body alignment (see Bicep Curl).

2. Extend your arm straight up above your head. Slightly bend your elbows but *do not lock them*. Your upper arms should be aligned with your ears (see Figure 7.103).

3. Exhale and bring the weight down in back of your head. Inhale and lift arms up. Do not lock your elbow.

4. Practice one set of eight. Rest, breathe, and repeat only if you feel well enough to do so.

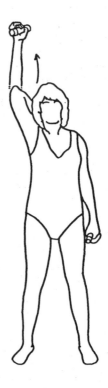

Figure 7.103 Tricep Extension

Cautions and Comments

- Do not exceed sixteen repetitions, making sure that you breathe properly.
- If raising your arms and hands above your head makes you dizzy, stop at once.
- In the later months of pregnancy, raising your arm in this fashion may cause dizziness or numbness. Stop if it does.

POSITIVE PREGNANCY FITNESS WET

Water is the natural environment in which your baby grows and develops. Spending some time in water yourself can help you to better understand just how your baby feels and perhaps make you feel even closer to your baby. Most pregnant women are attracted to the water, for it represents letting go, relaxation, and peace. During pregnancy you may want to relax in a nice, warm tub of water, for it will surely help you to relax and open up.

Swimming is often considered one of the best sports for pregnancy. The water supports your body weight, minimizes stress on your tissues and ligaments, and cools you as you exercise. In addition, swimming strengthens the abdominal and back muscles, thereby reducing the probability of backache in late pregnancy. Kicking promotes circulation and can help prevent or minimize varicose veins. Water acts as a resistance to muscular activities and so you can get a better but shorter workout than on dry land. You expend far less energy because the water acts as a buffer to create buoyancy. Being physically fit tends to help your baby, too. Your body works more efficiently and is better able to avoid an anaerobic or oxygen-depleted state. This means more oxygen available for your baby.

If you are not a swimmer, simply stretching at the shallow end of the pool can be enjoyable. Just being in warm, soothing water and focusing in on the sensations is very satisfying and pleasurable. Try moving slowly and enjoying the feeling of the water on your body as you breathe slowly and deeply with "Rock the Baby" breath (see page 19) in order to build up your strength and confidence.

Things to Remember

Make sure that there is a certified Red Cross lifeguard (ALS) or Red Cross Water Safety Instructor (WSI) present. You should also have the full permission of your health care professional in order to participate in any aquatic activity. *Never* go into the water if your amniotic sac has broken or you are experiencing vaginal bleeding. Just do those activities that you are comfortable with. You need not submerge yourself in the water if you don't want to. Try to tailor your program of water activities to the ones you enjoy the most.

You should alternate periods of activity with a stretching float so that all your muscles get a great workout without fatigue or cramping. Because of the aquatic support to your back, legs, and abdomen, you should not experience any backaches or round ligament cramps. Your routine should last 20-30 minutes and be done as often as possible, although even one session per week can make a measureable difference. The optimum water temperature for Moms-to-be is between 78° and 82° F. If you want to have a moderate swim, it is wise to do this before the PPF Wet routine. Good swimmers who wish to swim laps would be advised to do them moderately in order not to deplete the uterus of oxygen.

THE PPF WET PROGRAM *

---

1. Leg Lifts and Circles

Benefits

- Loosen entire pelvic area.
- Tone and keep legs shapely.
- Help drain excess blood from legs.

Directions

1. Stand in waist-high water. Hold onto the side of the pool with your right hand. Lift your left leg, flexing foot. Lower the leg. Do 5-8 lifts, relaxing the hips.

2. Lift your left leg up into the water and do 5-8 feet circles—flex the foot forward, to the side, back toward the knee and to the other side (see Figure 7.104).

3. Repeat on other side.

Cautions and Comments

- Do only small circles, since the resistance adds to the effort that you expel.
- You can also practice full leg circles to the right and to the left.

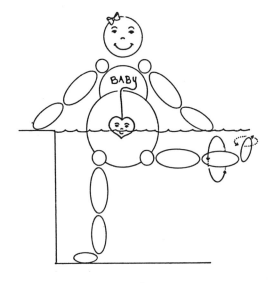

Figure 7.104   Leg Lifts and Circles

---

*Special thanks to Mary Grady, PPF Master Teacher, who created the PPF Wet Program. You can write to her at: 9736 Laurel Pine Dr., Richmond, VA 23228.

2. Knee Cradles

Benefits

- •Stretch the groin area.
- •Tone the thigh and buttocks muscles.

Directions

1. Hold the side of the pool with right hand. Bend your left knee, and hold with left hand. Stretch knee in and out to the side (see Figure 7.105).

2. Turn and repeat on other side.

Cautions and Comments

- •If you can't hold onto your foot, hold onto your calf or knee instead.

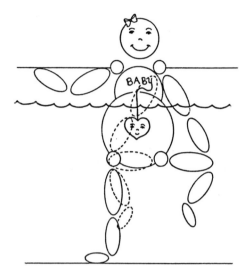

Figure 7.105 Knee Cradles

3. Side Stretch

Benefits

- •Keeps sides and waist toned.
- •Lifts rib cage off the diaphragm, thus making breathing easier.

Directions

1. Stand an arm's length from the pool, holding on with your right hand (see Figure 7.106). Bring left arm over head and bend at waist. Stretch left arm as close to the poolside as is comfortable.

2. As your left arm is coming over, swing the left hip out to the left side. As arm swings back, let the right hip swing

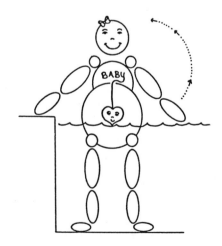

Figure 7.106 Preparing for Side Stretch

toward the pool (see Figure 7.107). Stretch for thirty seconds and return to the starting position.

3. Repeat on other side.

Cautions and Comments

- •The hip actions keep waist in tone and is a nice, graceful motion.
- •Closing your eyes and getting in tune with your body and baby really feels super.

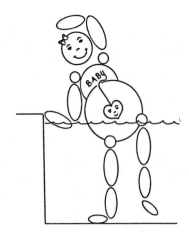

Figure 7.107   Side Stretch

4. Squats

Benefits

- •Stretch the gluteal muscles (buttocks), the hip adductors (groin), the quadraceps and thigh muscles.
- •Tone entire leg area and buttocks muscles.

Directions

1. Stand with your legs at least three feet apart. Hold the poolside with right hand. Fan the water with your left leg for added aerobic activity and toning (see Figure 7.108).

2. Bend your knees, feet pointing outward as far as is comfortable and pushing hips forward so as to keep the back straight. Hold for up to thirty seconds (see Figure 7.109).

3. Turn and repeat on other side.

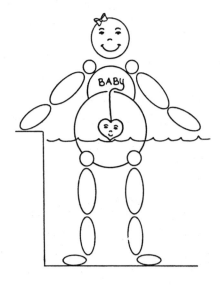

Figure 7.108   Position for Squats

Cautions and Comments

- •Although the water provides some support, remember to hold the side of the pool for balance.

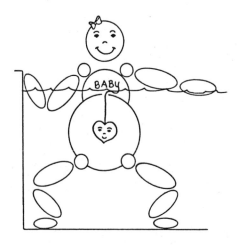

Figure 7.109 Squats

5. Pelvic Rocking

Benefits

- •Limbers the spine, making it flexible.
- •Helpful in eliminating or minimizing pregnancy backache.
- •Limbers and loosens the hips, the lumbar and pelvic attachments of the postvertebrals (erector spinae) and the abdominalis muscle group and the hip adductors (groin).

Directions

1. Stand straight with the knees slightly bent, legs a comfortable distance apart.

2. Exhale and tuck your pelvis forward. Your knees may bend a little more as your pelvis moves forward.

3. Inhale and straighten your back (see Figure 7.110).

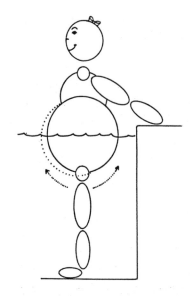

Figure 7.110 Pelvic Rocking

4. Repeat this pelvic rocking 5-10 times, coordinating your breathing with your pelvic movements.

Cautions and Comments

- Pelvic Rocking should be practiced every day to keep the lower torso area toned and flexible.
- Pelvic Rocking can be done during labor to help with back labor.

6. Practice Breath for Non-Swimmers

Benefits

- Acquaints non-swimmers with a reliable method of underwater breathing.
- Increases air capacity in the lungs.
- Reduces the non-swimmers' fear of submerging their faces.

Directions

1. Facing the pool wall, hold poolside with both hands.

2. Bring both feet up to the pool wall, placing them flat. Make sure the knees are bent.

3. Bring one knee up to each side of your baby area.

4. Inhale through the nose or mouth with your head up straight.

5. Tuck your chin to your neck so that your face is in the water and exhale through your nose. Keep your mouth closed.

Cautions and Comments

- The water and your arms will support you. Don't be afraid to pick up your feet.
- Exhaling through the nose will keep the water out of it. Make sure that your breathing is coordinated before you submerge your face.

7. Preparation for Baby Float

Benefits

- Gives you the feel of free floating underwater.
- Helps you to tune into your baby by being submerged in the same position as the baby is in.
- Enables you to practice the underwater breath.

Directions

1. Face the pool wall, holding on with both hands.

2. Place your feet flat on the pool wall with knees bent. Inhale (see Figure 7.111).

3. Tuck your chin and exhale in the water.

4. As you are exhaling, push off the wall with your feet and hold onto your knees (see Figure 7.112).

5. Float in the fetal position for about ten seconds, then bring your feet down and stand up.

Cautions and Comments

- Only do this in waist-high water.
- Don't be alarmed if you feel as though you are sinking—your body is very buoyant and will float up to the surface.
- Remember to exhale through your nose as long as your face is submerged.

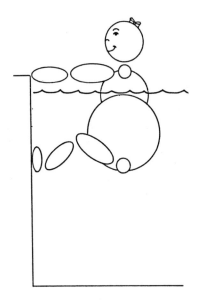

Figure 7.111 Preparation for Baby Float

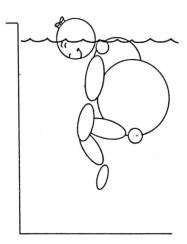

Figure 7.112 Practicing the Baby Float

8. Baby Float

Benefits

- Enables you to bond prenatally with your baby in the same environment and position as the baby.
- Maintains body coordination.
- Loosens and revitalizes the entire body.

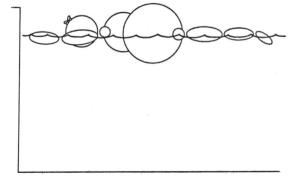

Figure 7.113   All Stretched Out in the Baby Float

Directions

1. You can either begin by holding onto the pool as in the previous exercise or by squatting down and grabbing the knees. Remember to blow out of your nose.

2. Lying forward in a fetal position, try to feel the way your baby must feel. Float for 5-10 seconds.

3. Release the knees, let your arms stretch over your head, and push your legs back in a prone position. Really feel that full body stretch (see Figure 7.113).

4. In one movement grab your knees again, lift your head, and take a breath. You can float in the Baby Float position (see Figure 7.114).

5. Lie back, stretching your arms over your head, and push legs forward (supine position).

6. Grab the knees, once more bringing the head up and legs down. Bring feet to the pool floor and stand.

7. Take two "Rock the Baby" breaths (see page 19).

Cautions and Comments

- Practice this in segments before trying to do the series all the way through.
- Remember to use your imagination while practicing the Baby Float. Get to know how your baby feels.

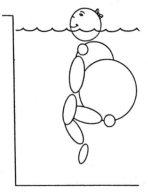

Figure 7.114   Breathing in the Baby Float

9. Arm Toners

Benefits

- Keep the arm muscles and shoulders toned and flexible.
- Expand the chest.
- Prepare the arms for the extra "baby things" you will soon have to carry.

Directions

1. Stand straight in the water, legs slightly apart.

2. Hold a plastic plate (about eight inches in diameter) in each hand. The plates will cause resistance.

Curls: Bring your arms in front of you, hands down at your thighs. Bend your elbows, bringing the arms up in front of you. Repeat 5-8 times (see Figure 7.115).

Side Lifts: Begin with your hands at your sides. Have your thumb on the flat part of the plate facing outward. Lift arm straight out to the side. Return your arm to the side by turning the plate sideways so that it is not resisting water coming down (see Figure 7.116). Repeat five times, then turn the thumb down and repeat five more times.

Cautions and Comments

- When returning the plate through the water during the Side Lifts, do so sideways, making a cutting motion through the water so as to reduce returning resistance.

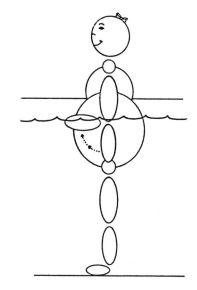

Figure 7.115 Curls

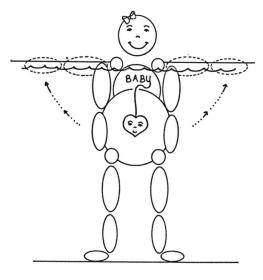

Figure 7.116 Side Lifts

10. Butterfly and "V" Stretch

Benefits

- •Stretches the perineal (pelvic floor) area, the hip adductors (groin), and the quadraceps.
- •Tones thigh and calf areas.
- •Tones arm and shoulder areas.

Directions

1. Place yourself in deep water.

2. With your back to the wall, hold onto the edge of the pool.

3. Bring the soles of your feet together and draw both feet up as close to the body as is comfortable.

4. Separate your feet and extend both legs out as far to either side as possible 4-6 times (see Figure 7.117).

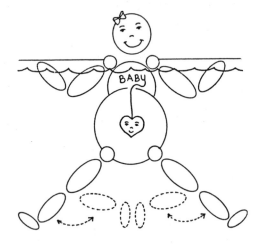

Figure 7.117   Butterfly/"V" Stretch

Cautions and Comments

- •If you can't swim, try this in shallow water. Your feet will touch the bottom but you will still experience the stretch.

11. Pendulum Legs

Benefits

- •Tone the waist, leg, arm, and abdominal areas.
- •Prepare the abdominal oblique muscles for the pushing stage of labor.
- •Gently strengthen the lower back.

Directions

1. Place yourself in deep water.

2. Face the pool wall. Put your elbows and forearms on the pool edge.

3. Keeping your upper body straight, move both legs to the right so that they are at about a 4 o'clock angle from your head. Swing them back down and to the left at the same angle. Repeat 4-6 times (see Figure 7.118).

Cautions and Comments

- If you are uncomfortable in deep water, don't do this exercise.
- If your baby area is not comfortable next to the wall, hold your body so it is not touching it.
- Do not try to lift your legs too far on either side.

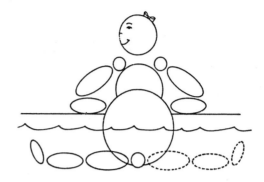

Figure 7.118 Pendulum Legs

12. Cooling Down

Benefits

- Brings the cardiovascular system down to a slower, non-active rate.
- Bonds and gets you in tune with your baby.
- Promotes deep relaxation.

Directions

1. Walk gracefully through the water, slowly swinging your arms.

2. Float either on your stomach or back. You may be surprised at how much more buoyant you are! The amniotic fluid that surrounds your baby enables you to float better.

Cautions and Comments

- Always cool down after any activity, especially if you do an aerobic activity.
- Because your body seems so much lighter in the water, you may feel like your old, slim self again!
- You can float for as long as you like; the water is very relaxing!

Other PPF exercises that can be practiced in the pool are:

- Hip Rotator (page 106)
- Standing Half Bow (page 113)

POSTPARTUM EXERCISES

If you start practicing the PPF program early in pregnancy and work with it throughout, you won't have fitness problems once you deliver your baby. I have devised the following practice schedules for both pregnancy and postpartum.

PRACTICE SCHEDULES

During Pregnancy

You should practice the following exercises 20-30 minutes every day or every other day:

- •"Rock the Baby" Breath (page 19)
- •The Basic Nine (page 71)
- •The Salute to the Child (page 94)
- •Complete Relaxation with Visualizations (page 158)
- •Any other PPF exercise you desire

During the Last Six Weeks of Pregnancy

You should practice the following exercises for 20-30 minutes, preferably with your birth assistant.

- •Breathing for Birth breaths: 10-15 minute practice session; practice each breath so that you can comfortably do it for 60-90 seconds
- •Complete Relaxation (page 158)
- •Various positions for labor and birth; hold each position for 1-3 minutes (page 205)
- •The Salute to the Child (page 94)
- •Any other PPF exercise you desire

During the First Three Weeks Postpartum

You should practice the following exercises beginning immediately after the baby's birth. Try to practice some of them while you take care of the baby.

Exercises After a Vaginal Delivery:

- Pelvic Floor Exercises (page 89)
- Abdominal Breath (page 89)
- Complete Relaxation lying on your tummy (page 158)
- Anal Lock in the shower (page 45)
- Baby Curls (#6 of the Basic Nine; page 86)
- Pregnancy Spinal Twist (#3 of the Basic Nine; page 76)
- Single Leg Lifts: Lying flat on your back, take ten seconds to lift one leg straight up into the air. Hold it up for ten seconds. Slowly lower it to the mat taking 15-20 seconds. Take 1-2 deep breaths. Repeat on other side. Do three more times.
- Head to Knee Pose: Lying flat on your back, lift one leg straight up. Bend the leg onto your chest and wrap your arms around the knee. Bring your forehead to your knee and hold for thirty seconds to two minutes. Lower the head, release the arms, straighten and lower the leg slowly, using the abdominal muscles. Repeat on other side. Do three more times.

Exercises After a Cesarean Birth:

- "Rock the Baby" Breath (page 19)
- The Bridge (#4 of the Basic Nine; page 81)
- Baby Curls (#6 of the Basic Nine; page 86)
- Side Leg Raises: Roll onto your side and put all your weight on your arms so you don't strain your abdominals. Begin raising your leg only a few inches above the bed. Increase this distance until your leg is all the way up into the air. Do 5-10 with each leg. *Don't lie on your back and raise your legs, for that would be too taxing on your surgery site.*
- Curl Backs (page 78)

Now that you have your baby, strictly follow the good posture directions on page 69. After 21-28 days your abdominal muscle tone will return and you can resume a regular exercise program. Try to exercise with your baby every day. Happy practicing!

Part II
Labor and Birth

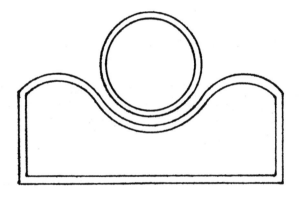

Ancient Egyptian symbol of birth

CHAPTER EIGHT
Complete Relaxation Self-Taught

The most important skill necessary for active participation in the birth process is the ability to relax at will. Most people do not fully understand the training that is needed to acquire this skill.

In this country, we do *things* to relax. We play tennis, we do needlepoint, we watch television, we read, etc. We usually call these *things* forms of relaxation. Actually, these things are activities which we enjoy doing, so we only *think* of them as forms of relaxation.

From a PPF point of view, the only effective form of relaxation is a body that is at rest and consciously relaxed. You may be thinking that this describes what you do every night when you go to sleep. But there is one major difference between relaxation and sleep. When you fall off to sleep, you are no longer conscious. When you learn to do a Complete Relaxation, you keep your awareness.

The best and most effective way to learn progressive relaxation is to practice it over and over again. It is an acquired skill which takes time, practice, and patience to develop. By continually commanding and allowing the body to relax, you will become totally familiar with this state of being. Once you have mastered this skill, you can use it in a variety of different situations. When you are in active labor, you can consciously enter this state at will between contractions, thereby saving your energy for the coming contraction. This same skill is invaluable if you are nursing your baby. Your physical relaxation will enable your milk to let down and will make the nursing experience more pleasurable and successful for both you and the child.

As you grow larger, you may find it more and more difficult to find comfortable positions. For that reason, a variety of suggested relaxation positions have been included. Try to choose and use only one position when you practice Complete Relaxation. If you give yourself the option of changing positions, you may spend the entire time shifting from one position to another rather than practicing relaxation. Try a Complete Relaxation at least once in each of the following positions to familiarize yourself with how each position feels.

Relaxation Using a Wall or Chair

Benefits

•Is a very easy position to relax in.
•Evenly distributes your body weight.

Directions

1. Sit on a soft mat, arranging pillows in back of you and underneath your legs.

2. Allow your head to be supported by the pillow or the chair behind you and make sure that your head is centered (see Figures 8.1 and 8.2).

3. Rest your hands on the baby area.

4. Let your feet rest a comfortable distance apart.

Cautions and Comments

•It is not advisable to rest flat on your back during pregnancy. As your uterus becomes larger and your baby becomes heavier, there is pressure on the blood vessels rising from the legs up along your backbone toward your heart. The weight of the pregnancy may block the flow enough to cause low blood pressure and dizziness. Or it can have the opposite effect, and decrease the blood flow to your kidneys so much that you respond by raising your blood pressure high above normal levels.

•Resting in a chair or using a wall is recommended for about the first five months of pregnancy. From then on, resting on your left side is strongly recommended.

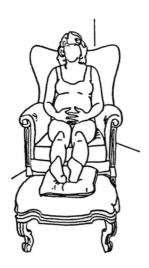

Figure 8.1 Relaxing in a Chair

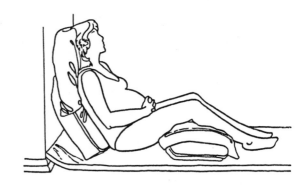

Figure 8.2 Relaxing Against a Wall

Side-Lying Relaxation Pose

Benefits

- Provides increased comfort in the later and larger months of pregnancy.
- Enables the body to completely relax.
- Frees the spine from bearing any weight so that it can be relaxed.
- Is an excellent sleeping position during the later months.

Directions

1. Lie on your left side, which is beneficial for your blood circulation. Place one pillow under your head and another one next to your legs on the inside. Bend your top knee and place it on the second pillow.

2. Place your hands in any comfortable position (see Figure 8.3). Placing a pillow between your legs takes the strain off your lower back (see Figure 8.4).

Cautions and Comments

- This is the most popular reclining position during the later months of pregnancy.

- You may want to add a third pillow near the middle of your back for extra comfort, or move the pillow near the legs up so that it fits under your abdomen. A pillow under the abdomen releases tension from the lower back.
- This is a popular breastfeeding position if you want to feed your baby while lying down.

The following posture, Complete Relaxation, may seem very simple to you as you read over the directions. You may think, "Oh, that's easy. This should be a snap to learn." Let me warn you before you begin that practicing this posture will take a lot of mental concentration. Your brain will try to divert you with more interesting tidbits and gossip. Don't get lost in your own idle thoughts while you try to practice this relaxation. If a thought comes in, let it pass; do not dwell on it as you then get back to the many steps involved in learning how to relax your body at will. With consistent mental and physical practice, you will master this all-important pose. Mastery of it will contribute to a more positive pregnancy, birth, and motherhood experience.

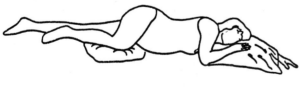

Figure 8.3 Left Side-Lying Position

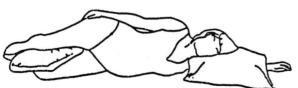

Figure 8.4 Pillow Between the Legs in a Left Side-Lying Position

Complete Relaxation

Benefits

- Deeply relaxes the muscles and nervous system.
- Releases stored tensions and anxieties, thereby restoring a peaceful feeling to the body and mind.
- Twenty minutes of Complete Relaxation is equal to two hours of sleep.
- Is a useful energizer.
- Prepares the pregnant woman for the relaxation periods between contractions.
- Helps to keep blood pressure within normal range.

Directions for Variation I: Contract, Release, Relax

1. Settle into a comfortable relaxation position.

2. Take 2-4 "Rock the Baby" breaths (see page 19) to get centered.

3. Close your eyes. Contract all the facial muscles. Try to move all the facial muscles toward the nose and feel the tightness. Hold for five seconds. Release. Breathe.

4. Squeeze the shoulders up around your neck and feel the tightness. Squeeze harder. Hold for five seconds. Release. Breathe.

5. Make fists with the hands and tighten the arms. Tighten harder as you raise them a few inches. Hold for five seconds. Release. Breathe.

6. Push the shoulder blades together. Squeeze harder. Hold for five seconds. Release. Breathe.

7. Contract the buttocks and feel the tightness. Squeeze harder. Hold for five seconds. Release. Breathe.

8. Tighten the thighs, knees, and calves. Feel the tightness. Hold for five seconds. Release. Breathe.

9. Push your heels away from the body by pointing the toes toward the knees as you feel the tightness. Hold for five seconds. Release. Breathe.

10. Open your mouth wide as you inhale and sigh out the breath: aaah. Repeat five times.

11. Focus your concentration on your facial muscles and feel the forehead and eyebrow area going limp. Let go of that area even more.

12. Mentally focus on your eyes. Relax them.

13. Feel your jaw muscles and cheek muscles let go. Feel the looseness. Separate your teeth and let your tongue fall back slightly into your mouth. Feel the muscles in the mouth area letting go.

14. Feel your nostrils, ears, and scalp relaxing.

15. Let all expression melt from your face. Feel it going limp.

16. Relax the neck: the front, the sides, the back.

17. Feel your shoulders letting go: the right shoulder, the left shoulder, and the space between.

18. Feel your upper arms, elbows, and lower arms relaxing.

19. Feel your fingers opening slightly and releasing.

20. Feel your chest and back going limp. Feel the top half of your body completely relaxed and loose.

21. Relax the tummy area to give the baby more room. Feel the inner abdominal muscles letting go.

22. Feel your buttocks going limp, letting go.

23. Focus in on the birth canal area and feel it loose and relaxed. Check to see that your mouth is still relaxed. Relax the mouth and the birth canal.

24. Feel your thighs, hips, knees, calves, and ankles going limp.

25. Feel your feet letting go. Let your toes relax one by one.

26. Take a moment or two to check your body over for further tension.

27. Feel yourself sinking into the mat or the chair. Let go, give up. Feel a sense of looseness enveloping you.

28. Feel the tensions draining out of your fingers and toes. Imagine a flow of tensions, tiredness, troubles, fears, anxieties, and aches leaving your body as you open all the muscles.

29. Let your breathing settle down to a comfortable rate as you sink into the blissful feeling of complete relaxation.

30. Allow your consciousness and your baby's consciousness to connect. Be receptive to any feelings from your child.

31. Try to keep your mental awareness on your child as you relax for 10-20 minutes.

32. When coming out of a Complete Relaxation, take your time.

33. First focus your awareness on how your body feels. Become aware of your hands and legs. Move your fingers slowly, then your toes, then begin to stretch and slowly come back to reality.

34. Walk yourself up into a sitting position using your hands if you are practicing lying down.

35. You should feel revitalized and reenergized after your practice.

Directions for Variation II: Release, Relax

1. Once you have mastered Variation I and find that you can relax your muscles at will, you can eliminate the muscle contraction part of this exercise.

2. You can begin your practice with #10.

Cautions and Comments

• This posture is much easier if someone else with a soothing voice reads the directions to you. Your husband or a friend may be able to help you out, or you can tape the directions for practicing.

• Do not be discouraged if it takes you a full twenty minutes just to get all your muscles to relax. Keep practicing until your body responds to your mental commands.

•Try not to fall asleep during this relaxation. Rather, go into a deep relaxation or a light meditative state with mental clarity.

•See Chapter 9 for a variety of topics on which to mentally focus when you practice Complete Relaxation.

•See the Appendix for information regarding my *Relax and Enjoy Your Baby Within* practice tape.

CHAPTER NINE
Prenatal Psychology and "Inner Bonding"

Have you ever wondered what your baby is thinking as it develops inside you? Emotional and psychological development in utero has been debated for many years. Not until the advent of ultrasound technology have we been able to actually see the unborn's reaction to pain, touch, and reflex activity—things that were previously considered underdeveloped at birth. Today, many professionals in medicine and psychology are actively studying prebirth consciousness, and their findings may surprise you. The womb is finally beginning to be seen as more than just a place for physical maturation. It is also a place of mental and emotional growth.

Dr. Thomas Verny, a Canadian psychiatrist, is an avid researcher in the field of pre- and peri-natal psychology. In his book, *The Secret Life of the Unborn Child*, he relates some surprising findings relating to the environment in the womb. His book not only deals with the phenomena of the unborn, but also discusses the effect of language, music, and other environmental factors on the fetus in utero and into early childhood. Through Dr. Verny's research and other pioneering work in this new field, we are beginning to discover that the unborn child is more advanced (both emotionally and mentally) than we ever suspected.

Following is a condensed summary of some of the findings:

- By the fourth month, the unborn will suck if its lips are stroked. If a bitter substance like iodine is introduced into the amniotic fluid, it will grimace and refuse to swallow the liquid. But if a sweet substance like saccharine is introduced, it will double its normal rate of ingestion.
- By the fourth month, the unborn begins to suck its thumb and grasp and play with its umbilical cord.

- By the fourth month, if a bright light is projected onto the mother's abdomen, the baby will gradually move its tiny hands up toward its eyes. If a loud noise is made, the unborn will raise its hands and cover its ears.
- By the sixth month, the unborn's hearing system is completely developed. Because water is a better conductor of sound than air, the baby can hear very well, although distorted.
- By the seventh month, recordings of the baby's brain waves show that during sleep the baby exhibits Rapid Eye Movements (REM). In adults, REM sleep is almost always associated with dreaming. Therefore, it is logical to conclude that babies must dream by the seventh month. The unborn child is also keyed into the mother's heartbeat. Violent shifts of the unborn's body or variations in heartbeat signal the unborn's discomfort or experience of stress.
- By the seventh month, the unborn is able to "play" with its parents through the abdominal wall. If you gently push with one finger into your abdomen, first on one side and then on the other, your baby will eventually pick up on the game and start pushing back.

THE WORLD OF THE UNBORN CHILD

Research indicates that within the first three months of life, the tiny embryo can bend its neck, trunk, pelvis, and pull its arms and legs away from the body. Swallowing occurs at twelve weeks, gag reflex and tastebuds function at fourteen weeks, hearing at twenty weeks, and sucking at twenty-two weeks. By twenty-four weeks, the fetus is capable of floating peacefully, kicking, turning somersaults, hiccoughing, urinating, sighing, swallowing, becoming excited at sudden noises, and calming down when the mother talks. From the fourth month on there is the capacity for conditioned learning and, therefore, rudimentary memory and intentional behavior. During the fifth month the unborn experiences periods of drowsiness and sleep alternated with periods of activity, and can discriminate differences in sounds. By the seventh month the unborn can move in rhythm to music and even shows a definite preference for some kinds of music.

INCREASING AWARENESS IN THE UNBORN

After reading about your unborn baby's capabilities, you might want to increase its awareness even more. There are a number of very simple exercises that may be included in your prenatal program to stimulate, teach, and nurture your unborn baby.

Visualizations for ''Inner Bonding''

Relaxing visualizations (see the end of this chapter) put you in tune with your baby and allow you to pick up on the baby's subtle movements and sounds. During a concentration, there is actual communication between you and your baby. In a relaxed state, your emotions and thinking processes are increased and more sensitive to these subtle changes. If you really listen to your baby, you will feel increased movements. This is sometimes due to an increase in oxygen. In actuality, your baby is tuning into your increased attention.

Talking

Talking to your baby from the very beginning is a wonderful means of contact not only for you, but for the whole family. Each family member has a different voice, and your unborn child will respond to the different vibrations. Fathers especially enjoy talking to the baby every day. Reading aloud to your unborn baby is an excellent idea. Explaining your dreams to the baby (after all, he or she was *there*!) is also a good idea.

Eventually you will begin to see your unborn baby as a tiny person with thoughts, feelings and even a personality. Talking is an excellent way for your other children to begin to develop a sibling relationship and be included in prenatal care as well.

Touching

Touching your unborn child gives you a real sense of the "someone" growing inside you. Your husband or your other children will become more comfortable touching your abdomen. You can trace the baby's shape. Look for arms, legs, head, and feet. Make it a family affair. Children love to trace what they think the baby looks like using a washable pen. The *kind* of touch is important, too. Unborn babies do not like sharp pokes or fast rubbing and much prefer gentle stroking, soft pats, and rubs. You can do "effleurage" (gentle massage strokes) on your abdomen or you can massage it with oil. Use a soft nerf ball and roll it around on your tummy to create a new sensation for your unborn child.

When tracing body outlines, your baby may respond by curling up in one part of the uterus. If you gently stroke its back, the body will relax again and extend its arms and legs.

Practicing Parenting Skills

Some mothers are overly concerned that "everything I do will affect the baby" or "I have to do it perfectly." Just remember that fleeting worries or anxieties are a normal part of pregnancy. They have no adverse effects on the baby. Only deep, persistent, negative feelings can cause harm to your baby. Just be yourself. Being more in touch with this new little person and its inner world can add intimacy and a deep sense of bonding before birth. *Love Chords*, a cassette tape produced by Dr. Thomas Verny and Sandra Collier, stimulates and enhances the emotional and intellectual development of your unborn child. (For further information on the benefits of this beautiful tape and how to order, see the Appendix.)

Preparing Yourself Through Visualization

The exercise segments of the PPF program explain the many physiological changes that occur during pregnancy and birth and how you can work with these changes to ensure more comfort and ease in your pregnancy. Visualization can help you to integrate your mind and body. In essence, you can learn to program your mind for optimum health and well-being. You can prepare yourself for your upcoming birth experience by discovering your own inner strengths and your capacity to love your unborn baby as it grows.

Bonding: Meeting Your Baby

Within the last few years some practitioners in the medical community have begun to realize the vital role that bonding plays in the parent-child relationship. Bonding refers to the first minutes and hours spent with your new baby right after birth. The emotional tie that develops during this time has a very positive effect on the relationship between parents and child in future years.

Because your baby's consciousness is already developing while you are inwardly-oriented during pregnancy, you can practice a pleasant form of "inner bonding" at this time, too. To encourage mental preparation for your baby's birth, some very enjoyable visualizations have been developed.

Using your imagination to create different scenes and experiences, often including your future child, forms the basis of the following mental visualization exercises. These mental trips will strengthen the tie with your child and teach you how to control your brain. Although it takes some mental effort to experience the following visualizations, the time spent disciplining your brain will produce tangible rewards: peace of mind, a positive mental attitude, and, most importantly, a warm anticipation of your new and future child.

Scientists have recently been studying what babies sense and how they feel emotionally while inside the womb. The latest conclusion, based on exhaustive study, is that babies are in a state of euphoria during the developmental time inside. All their bodily needs are taken care of by the mother's body, leaving the infant free to experience movement, sounds, feelings, intuition, and bliss. By practicing Complete Relaxation in conjunction with visualization, you can learn how to share in your baby's bliss. Although your body automatically provides for your baby, your consciousness must be trained to mentally link with your child.

The following visualizations for optimum health and well-being should be used in combination with Complete Relaxation. It is only in a relaxed state that you can really delve into visualization and thoroughly enjoy it. If you haven't yet practiced Complete Relaxation (pp. 158-159), take the time to do so before trying any of the following visualizations. You will find that it takes inner determination to mentally complete a visualization. If your mind wanders while you are practicing, immediately bring your attention back to the exercise. You may have to practice each exercise several times in order to do it from beginning to end. Having someone else read the instructions to you may be quite helpful. If you make a Complete Relaxation tape for yourself, you can easily add any one of these visualizations to it. See the Appendix for information regarding *Relax and Enjoy Your Baby Within,* an already-made tape.

Visualizations for "Inner Bonding"

The Baby's Birth Trip

1. Do a Complete Relaxation (pp. 158-159).

2. Take 2-3 "Rock the Baby" breaths (see page 19) to center yourself and bring your awareness to your child.

3. Concentrating on your baby, use your imagination and pretend that you are the baby for a few moments.

4. Imagine how your baby feels— warm, wet, quite contented and blissful. Become the baby as you imagine your arms and legs tightly closed next to you. Feel the softness of the conforming walls all around you.

5. Imagine the regular thumping of the blood pulsing by. Hear the other noises surrounding this warm, compact home.

6. Suddenly begin to feel the soft walls getting harder and squeezing you, then squeezing you even harder. Then they are released and everything is back to normal.

7. Continue to feel the walls tightening around you, squeezing you again, but for a longer period of time. "When will this end?" you are thinking. Then the squeezing stops only to begin again.

8. Now there is a new sensation: a feeling of great pressure from behind— pushing, pushing, pushing even harder.

9. You are being pushed down a narrow, dark, warm tunnel. Feel yourself being pushed forcefully down, only to slide back up again. In your consciousness hear your mother reassuring you that she is with you and will protect you. Feel another push and great pressure behind you.

10. Sense that this black tunnel has an opening and you are getting near to it, as you feel great pressure on your face. Hear another message from your mother saying this trip is almost over.

11. Finally, with great force, your head is pushed through the end of the tunnel into a new place. It is bright, there are new noises. Feel some pressure on your head as someone touches it and guides you out.

12. Feel several more strong pushes as you are squeezed out of the tunnel. Feel warm hands holding you.

13. All of a sudden there is a warm, soft place below you and you can hear that familiar heartbeat once again. It reminds you of the place you used to be in.

14. Feel warm, protected, and loved on your mother's tummy. Be thankful that the birth trip is over.

15. Now shift your concentrations away from that imaginary trip to your baby inside, who is going to make a similar trip very soon.

16. Reassure your child that you will be there with him or her throughout the birth trip. You will be waiting expectantly to meet, love, hold, and cuddle this new baby. Mentally discuss this and other feelings with your child for a few moments.

17. Rouse yourself when you find your mind drifting.

18. Wiggle your fingers and feel them move, just as your baby inside feels his or her fingers move. Feel your toes moving. Stretch and feel your feet just as your baby does.

19. Return to your former level of awareness with a better understanding of what is coming for your child and the very vital role you will play in this experience.

CAUTION: This visualization should only be practiced during the last six weeks of pregnancy. (Available in the *Breathing for Birth* tape; see the Appendix.)

The Golden Ray of Sunshine

1. Do a Complete Relaxation (page 158) until you are relaxed in a comfortable position.

2. Imagine that you are lying on a white beach on your own special island. This island is a magical place where all kinds of wonderful things can happen.

3. Feel a special golden ray of sunshine shining down on you. This sunshine will not burn you in any way. It has healing, tension-releasing, and rejuvenating powers.

4. Feel the sunshine on your outer body. Feel it on your face, your chest, your arms, your fingers, your legs, and your feet.

5. Feel the warmth all over the baby area of your body.

6. Imagine this special sunshine going right through your skin and into your body.

7. Feel this healing light inside your head melting away your worries.

8. Feel this special light inside your chest, inside your arms, your hands, your legs, your feet, and your buttocks.

9. Feel this shiny golden light warming and preparing your birth canal area for the coming adventure.

10. Imagine this special light encircling your baby like a big golden bubble.

11. Bathe your baby in this golden bath of healing light.

12. Feel your whole being and that of your baby being energized.

13. Remain in this golden light for several moments. Enjoy its feelings of inner warmth and protection.

14. Rouse yourself slowly and deliberately when you want to get up. Take 1-2 deep breaths and slowly rouse your hands and feet, then the rest of your body.

Opening Up to Bliss

1. In any comfortable position, practice Complete Relaxation (see page 158) until you are fully relaxed.

2. Center your awareness on the baby growing inside you. See if you can feel the baby at this moment.

3. Now consciously quiet your mind by concentrating for several minutes on your breath coming in and going out. Let your breathing settle down.

4. Begin to dwell with your child as you imagine your whole being opening up to him or her.

5. Let the bliss, the contentment, the protection, the happiness, the love that your baby feels and lives with at this moment, pour into you.

6. Imagine a secret doorway through which these wonderful feelings can pass to you. Open the doorway a bit wider so that you can be flooded with these good and satisfying feelings.

7. Accept the fact that your child can give to you, just as you give and will continue to give to your child.

8. Immerse yourself in these good feelings for a few more moments.

9. Rouse yourself slowly and conscientiously to retain any remnant of these pleasurable feelings.

Sharing Your Baby's Present Home

1. Go through all the steps of a Complete Relaxation (p. 158).

2. Focus your mental awareness on a beautiful beach near a warm, calm body of water. Look around and notice all the details of the scene: the color of the sand or earth, the kind of trees, the color of the sky, the water.

3. Listen and hear some birds singing and chirping, hear the trees move in a slight warm wind, notice the flowers growing near the water.

4. Feel yourself becoming filled with a sense of security and protection as you dwell in your own special place. Feel a sense of ease, a letting go of tensions and worries.

5. Feel yourself walking on the warm, soft ground. There is nothing on the ground that can hurt you in any way. Feel your body walking slowly toward the water. Notice the weight of your body, its movement.

6. The water is so warm, pleasant, and clear as your feet enter it. It is the perfect temperature, and you can feel the soft, warm sand at the bottom. There is nothing in the water that can hurt or harm you in any way.

7. Feel your calves entering the water. Then your thighs and your torso, until you are finally standing up in the water submerged to your shoulders. The water is calm, warm, and comforting.

8. Splash some water on your face. Move your arms around under the water. Notice how easily you can move your arms, how light your body feels. How effortless it is to move! Feel the weightlessness of your body, your ease of movement in the water as your tiredness and tensions are washed away.

9. Take a few moments to either swim or to stand next to a warm waterfall that is cascading into the water. Feel protected, warmed, comforted, and cleansed by the water. Feel yourself filling up with contentment.

10. Become aware of your baby growing inside, who is feeling the very same way as you do at this moment.

11. Open yourself up to your child and let your feelings blend as you share your baby's home inside your body. Know that your baby is also protected and safe.

12. Remain in this pleasant state for several minutes. If a negative or distracting thought crosses your mind, simply let it go and return to the feelings in the warm water.

13. Focus on how you feel in the water as you begin to come out and back onto the land. The air is warm, so you will not be chilled. Feel your head coming out of the water, then your shoulders, then your arms and torso, and finally your legs. Your whole body is out of the water. Notice the effect of gravity on your body.

14. Notice the weight of your body as you slowly come out of the water. Notice that it takes more effort to move. A fluffy towel is nearby. Pick it up and dry yourself off.

15. Looking up, you notice a soft blanket. Lie down on the blanket and let the sun warm all those places inside you that were filled with tension, fatigue, and heaviness.

16. Let your body become a sponge absorbing the golden sunshine. The sun cannot burn or hurt you in any way. Feel it filling your head, your arms and shoulders, your chest, your back, your abdomen, your buttocks, your legs and feet. Feel the sunshine filling your baby inside with vitality and energy.

17. Notice how each part of your body feels. Notice your hands. Notice your arms, your lower back, the back of your head.

18. Notice what you are thinking about. Watch your thoughts roll by. Be an observer.

19. Become aware of your fingers again and begin to move the fingers on each hand very slowly. Make loose fists with your hands. Now open them. Repeat this several times.

20. Slowly wiggle your toes. Move your head from side to side. Slowly begin to return to this level of awareness. Begin to stretch luxuriously.

21. Take one or two minutes to completely reawaken. You will feel refreshed and renewed, and be in closer contact with your unborn baby.

CHAPTER TEN

The Physiology of Birth

Within the warm, dark, inner recesses of your being at one unnoticed moment in time, a new consciousness begins its journey into life. Conception is truly one of nature's miracles. Each month, an ovum (or mature egg) is released from your ovary. The egg must make a ten-day journey to the cavity of the uterus more than three inches away. The path that the egg must take is through the Fallopian tube, where the passageway at the inner end is no larger than a bristle. The ovum must make this journey without any means of locomotion. It must depend on external methods for propulsion. A stream of fluid, tiny hairlike projections, and the muscular motion of the Fallopian tube itself propels the tiny ovum toward the uterus. When the ovum is scarcely a third of the way down the tube, the grand event occurs: it meets a sperm and a new human being is begun! The genetic material of the father is added to that of the mother in fertilization. Immediately after fertilization, early cell division results in a solid ball of cells which resembles a raspberry and is called a "morula." This growth occurs within 96 hours after conception. Cell division continues and the cell mass develops two distinct regions: an outer layer of cells which will form the placenta, and an inner ball of cells which is the embryo and will become a fully developed baby. The cell mass implants itself into the uterine wall after a seven-day journey down the Fallopian tube and into the uterus. This is the time in the monthly cycle when the lining of the uterus has reached its greatest thickness. The nesting cluster of cells continues to multiply and transform rapidly. As the months progress the baby grows and develops. There are also some other changes occurring within your body that may surprise you:

- Your total blood volume increases from 30-60 percent during pregnancy.

- As a result, the heart has to pump fifty percent more blood per minute.

- The lungs are under pressure from the uterus, but your rib cage will widen to help compensate for this.

- The pregnant woman breathes much more air than the nonpregnant woman.

- The digestive system is not as efficient due to the growing uterus.

It should be obvious from these changes how beneficial controlled breathing and physical exercises can be during your pregnancy.

LABOR AND BIRTH

Labor is the climax of the maternity cycle. It is the process by which the fetus (baby) travels from the uterus to the outside world. This process begins with "lightening" and ends with the expulsion of the afterbirth or placenta.

Lightening

Tips and Other Information

- The baby descends lower into your pelvic area.
- After the baby has dropped, you may find it easier to breathe, but that urination is more frequent.
- You may walk around in this condition for several days or weeks.

How PPF Helps

- Keep practicing the PPF exercises, especially Salute to the Child (page 94), to keep your body in top shape for the impending birth.
- Increase your practice of Baby Breath (page 23) to facilitate the pushing part of labor.
- Practice the Breathing for Birth Breaths (page 199).
- Do a 15-20 minute Complete Relaxation (page 158) each day.

First Stage of Labor

Tips and Other Information

- The baby's head has moved more deeply into the pelvic outlet.
- The cervix has thinned and is beginning to dilate (see Figure 10.1). It must open a full ten centimeters (four inches) for this part of labor to be over.
- The cervix must open wide enough for your baby's head to be pushed out.

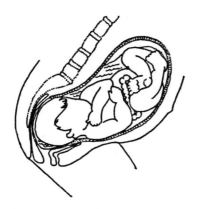

Figure 10.1 First Stage of Labor: Cervix is opened 5 cms.

How PPF Helps

- Use your PPF Breathing for Birth techniques (p. 199). Follow your birth assistant's directions.
- Use an outside focal point for concentration.
- Completely relax all voluntary muscles between contractions.
- Keep in mental contact with your baby via an inner dialogue. Offer reassurance that you will be there to hold and love the baby once the birth experience is over.

Transition: the Late First Stage of Labor

Tips and Other Information

- The cervix is nine centimeters dilated and the baby's head is beginning to rotate.
- You may be having irrational thoughts and feelings at this time. You may feel ready to give up, get very hot or very cold and possibly shaky.
- The baby will be born very soon!

How PPF Helps

- Continue to use your Breathing for Birth techniques (pg. 199).
- Pay strict attention to your birth assistant as the breathing rhythm is switched.
- Keep in mental contact with the baby (between contractions), who is also experiencing these strong contractions.
- Have birth assistant massage lower back to eliminate pain.
- Use Blowing Breath (page 202) if you have a premature urge to push.

Second Stage of Labor (Pushing)

Tips and Other Information

- The opening of the cervix is completed and you can begin to push through each contraction (see Figure 10.2).

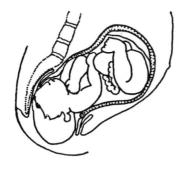

Figure 10.2 Second Stage of Labor: Pushing

- You may wonder where you get the energy for this pushing, but you will have it!

How PPF Helps

- All the squatting and pelvic loosening exercises will allow your pelvis to open its widest. Your child's head will fit so snugly that any bit of extra space will help you greatly at this time.
- If you have practiced your Baby Curls, it will pay off now.
- Use Pushing Breath (p. 203).
- Relax completely between pushes.

Crowning

Tips and Other Information

- As you push through each contraction, the baby's head will finally be delivered (see Figure 10.3).
- You may feel it as a burning and/or stretching sensation.

How PPF Helps

- You will need to use Blowing Breath (page 202) right after the baby has crowned to slow down the delivery of the rest of the child.

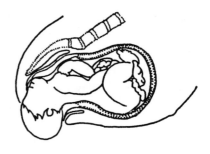

Figure 10.3 Crowning: The baby's head is born.

Rotation of the Head

Tips and Other Information

- After the birth of the baby's head, he or she will turn to one side without any help.
- This allows the shoulders to come out one at a time.
- Once the shoulders are out, the infant's body will quickly follow. See Figure 10.4.
- Keep your mental dialogue with the baby going throughout the final phases of birth.

How PPF Helps

- You will have to use Blowing Breath (page 202) to keep from pushing.

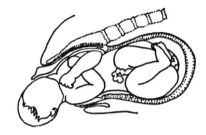

Figure 10.4 Rotation of the Head: Baby turns as shoulder is born.

Third Stage of Labor (Expulsion of the Afterbirth)

Tips and Other Information

- Pushing through several more contractions will expel the afterbirth.
- Afterbirth contractions also serve to reduce uterine hemorrhage.

How PPF Helps

- You will have to breathe and push through several more contractions.

- Make your mental dialogue a verbal one by welcoming your baby into the world!!

If you are faithful in your practice of PPF exercises, and breathing and relaxing techniques, your body will work beautifully for you and your baby.

CHAPTER ELEVEN
Massage and Pressure Points for Pregnancy, Labor, and Parenthood*

Massage can help to relax the body and increase circulation, sensation, and energy while promoting a general sense of well-being. (Not to mention the fact that it feels great!) Touching is a very powerful means of nonverbal communication between people. Massage can add new dimensions to the relationship between you and your mate. The type of massage described in this chapter can be used throughout the pregnancy, labor, and postpartum period. Massage during labor will depend on your own personal birth experience. Massage will help you to tune into your sensual self, and enable you to more clearly and vividly experience daily events in your life. This heightened sensitivity can add joy to your everyday life.

SOME SIMPLE RULES FOR MASSAGE

1. The receiver should choose a comfortable position that may change during the massage. Positions may also vary as the pregnancy progresses.

2. The time spent for massage will vary as the months go by. During early and mid pregnancy, 30-60 minutes will be enjoyable, whereas in the last few months, 15-45 minutes may be adequate.

---

*Special thanks to Charis Tondreau and David Engler, Certified Therapeutic Massage Therapists, and Grace Burkhardt, RN, New York City PPF Instructor, who helped in the preparation of this chapter.

3. When giving a massage, it is important to keep in mind: receiver's position, stroke pressure, and duration of each massage stroke. Ask the pregnant woman if there is a special tight spot that may be causing her tension, cramps, aches, etc. and needs to be worked on.

4. During the massage, check with the receiver now and then to see if she is experiencing any discomfort such as headache, nausea, or dizziness. If she is, stop massaging immediately and allow her to resume a more comfortable position.

5. Be sure to tune into the receiver's breathing. It should be relaxed and smooth. If it isn't, then work on relaxation techniques with the pregnant woman to develop a smooth and gentle breathing pattern.

6. When you are using different strokes during a massage, glide from one to the other as smoothly as you can.

7. Use more pressure when stroking toward the heart and less pressure when going away from the heart.

8. Try to mold your hands to your partner's contours.

9. Smoothly vary the speed and pressure of your strokes.

10. The person who is receiving the massage should be passive and should not try to help out during the massage. The receiver should have her eyes closed, thus promoting greater relaxation and enjoyment of the sensations.

11. Centering and tuning into the stroking sensations should be the receiver's main concern.

12. Too much massage in an irregular pattern and without lubrication—can actually make your partner more tense.

13. *Never* massage or use any pressure *directly on* the backbone (spine).

14. Keep in mind that a massage movement or technique should "feel" good to the giver, as well as the receiver.

15. *Never* massage a pregnant woman who has a full or empty stomach or is over-fatigued.

16. Avoid working on any skin surfaces that contain contusions, scars, or infections.

SPECIAL RESTRICTIONS FOR PREGNANT WOMEN

Women with varicose veins should receive only light, feather-like strokes on the legs. Their legs should also be elevated during a massage. Similarly, women who are suffering from hypertension, pre-eclampsia, or toxemia (heart trouble) should receive only very light massage.

The pregnant abdomen should only be very lightly massaged. *Never put pressure on it.* Women in the later months of pregnancy should *never* lie flat on their abdomens during a massage. *Do not massage* with a deep pressure around the ankles or on the inner ankles behind the tibia. Shiatsu Pressure Point Spleen 6 is located four finger lengths up from the inner ankle bone behind the tibia. This spot can trigger early or premature labor, so avoid it (see Figure 11.1).

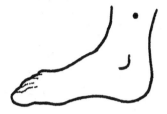

Figure 11.1   Avoid this pressure point throughout the pregnancy, but use during labor for any difficulties.

PREPARING FOR MASSAGE

1. Choose a warm, quiet place.

2. Massage on a carpeted floor. Spread out a blanket with an old sheet on top (in case you spill some oil). During the later months of pregnancy, it is often advantageous for the receiver to sit with her legs open facing the back of an armless chair, with her partner sitting in a chair facing her back (see Figure 11.2). The receiver may want to put her head on one or two pillows on top of the chair. Some women prefer to be massaged in a side-lying position with pillows under their head and abdomen. But this position may be quite uncomfortable for the person giving the massage. If it is agreeable to the giver, however, then this position can also be utilized. When using a side-lying position, half of the back is worked first and then the second half is massaged when the woman turns over.

3. Scented oil can be found in many health food stores, or you might try Almond Oil. *Never* use mineral oil because it removes the moisture from the skin. It is also wise not to use talc when doing a massage. Talc has been linked with lung cancer because the particles remain in the air, become inhaled, and damage the cilia (tiny hairs) in the respiratory tract. Tiger Balm (red or white) is good to use on sore muscles.

    Everyone absorbs oil differently. It is wise to begin with less oil, adding more if necessary. *Less* oil permits you to work deeper into the muscles; more oil is used for more superficial, soothing strokes. Use only a little oil on the face, hands, and feet.

    The oil enables your hands to apply pressure while moving smoothly over the surface of the skin. Store the oil in a squeeze bottle with a closeable top so it won't spill. Heat the bottle under hot water before using or squeeze some oil into your palm and rub your hands together to warm it. NOTE: *Vegetable oil will ultimately stain towels, so use old ones for massage.*

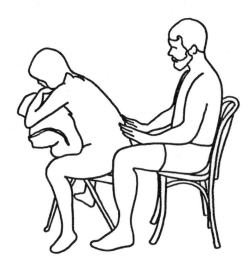

Figure 11.2 Late Pregnancy Position
for Massage

4. The person receiving the massage should be nude. Keep a sheet or light blanket handy in case the receiver gets cold. Keep the area not being worked on covered to prevent a chill.

5. Make sure your nails are short so you don't hurt your partner. Nails should be manicured to the level of the fingertip. Remove all hand jewelry, including watches.

6. Light a scented candle or some mild incense and put on soft music for a warm and relaxing atmosphere (see the Appendix for suggested massage music). Try to make the atmosphere as intimate and soothing as possible.

Massaging the Back and Shoulders

When to Use

This can be used during labor to induce relaxation.

Directions

1. Have the receiver get into a comfortable position (see Figure 11.2).

2. Begin to center by taking two or three "Rock the Baby" breaths (see page 19) together.

3. Squeeze some of the warmed oil onto your hands and rub them together until warm. Never pour oil directly on the person who is receiving the massage.

4. Place your palms on the lower back and slowly, with some pleasant pressure, move your hands up the shoulders on either side of the spine, across the shoulders, then back down along the sides of the back to

the starting point. Try to evenly cover the whole back area with oil. Look for tense areas while doing this motion. Repeat this stroke several times, trying to make the motions flow smoothly.

5. Place both wrists together on the lowest lumbar region of the spine (see Figure 11.3). Take a deep breath and, as you exhale, gently press into the lower back with your hands. Use your entire upper body for the movement, rather than just your hands. Check with your partner for a reaction. This area may need to be massaged particularly during back labor.

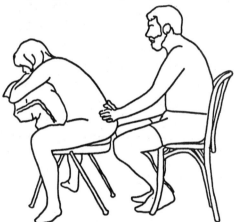

Figure 11.3 Hand-Massaging the Lowest Section of the Spine

The giver may find this movement tiring at first and will eventually begin to develop the muscles for a sustained massage. To relieve back labor, the birthing assistant can use flat hands, fists, two tennis balls, or even a small paint roller to apply lower back pressure. It is advisable for the birthing assistant to practice this part of the massage so you can become familiar with it and also because it can be quite tiring.

6. Once the lower back becomes somewhat relaxed, move your attention to the waist area. This is an area of extreme tension and pain during pregnancy. You should sit at a right angle to the receiver (see Figure 11.4). First oil your lower arms. Then, making fists, move one arm forward across the lower back, then the other in a sawing motion. Move your arms up and down the receiver's back slowly several times using this forward/backward motion (see Figures 11.4a and 11.4b).

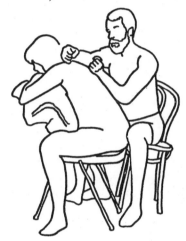

Figure 11.4a Sawing Motions Up the Spine

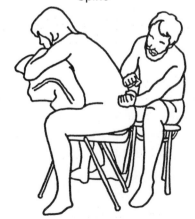

Figure 11.4b Sawing Motions Down the Spine

7. Facing your partner once again, place your thumbs in the grooves about 1/4"-1/2" on either side of the spine. Press firmly against the skin, using small, circular movements. Be sure to keep your thumbs in constant contact with the skin as you make little circles. If you find a sensitive spot or hard lump, have your partner breathe in deeply. As she exhales, have her imagine the breath flowing down to that spot. Upon exhalation press in with the thumb, very gradually, to go in a little bit deeper. This can be done two or three times in one spot. When pressing deeper remember to do it slowly and gradually, holding only 5-6 seconds each time. This technique can be used on all other parts of the body except the abdomen and near the ankles.

8. When your thumbs reach the top of the spine, place your index fingers on either side and gently (but firmly) move your fingers down on either side of the spine until they reach the buttocks. Repeat this three times.

9. Once you are ready to massage the neck and shoulder area (a high-tension area), place your thumbs between the upper back and lower neck. Using some pressure, make circles with your thumbs as you move to the sides of the neck. Concentrate on those areas that seem hard and firm. Work on these tight muscles until they loosen up.

10. Clasp one hand on top of a shoulder and pull back. Follow with the second hand in a hand-over-hand pulling motion (see Figure 11.5). Repeat this motion 5-10 times, then shift to

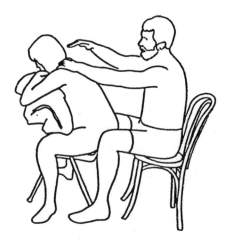

Figure 11.5 Massaging the Neck and Shoulder Areas

the other shoulder and massage it 5-10 times. When finished, place one hand on each shoulder and pull them back and then down the back to the buttocks. Use firm pressure as you move. (Keep in mind that inventing some of your own motions to share with your partner is a wonderful way to enhance a massage.)

11. Finish this massage with the nerve stroke. Lightly place your fingertips on top of your partner's head. Slowly and lightly move your fingers down the back—barely touching it—to the buttocks area. Repeat this light effleurage 3-4 times as a signal that the back massage is over. The nerve stroke helps to soothe and relax the nervous system. You may repeat this light effleurage all the way down the front of the inner thighs, down the inner legs, to the feet and toes. This allows the excess tension and energy to leave the body, enabling your partner to experience a feeling of lightness. This technique may be used particularly during labor—usually early and mid-labor.

Foot Massage

When to Use

Can be used during labor but feels fabulous anytime.

Directions

1. Have the receiver sit comfortably or lie down (see Figure 11.6) with the foot to be worked on resting on a cushion. Place one hand on the bottom part of the foot and the other hand on top of the foot. Pull down and off the foot as if you are "pulling" the tension out of the other person. Repeat 5-10 times on each foot. This motion is especially good during labor to pull some of the pain out of the body. You can have a nurse work on the other foot at the same time.

2. Place your thumbs on either ankle bone and gently circle each bone with firm pressure. Squeeze the achilles area (or back) of the foot gently. *Remember not to work higher than the ankle bone area.*

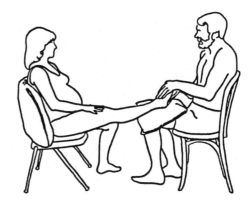

Figure 11.6   Foot Massage

3. Gently work the arch with your thumbs, applying firm pressure but using long strokes to cover the entire arch area.

4. Finish the foot massage with a stroke of your own invention. By the end of the day, Mom's feet are weary from carrying around her weight and the baby's, so spend a few moments "energizing" them.

PRESSURE POINTS TO USE DURING LABOR

Pressure point therapy can help during labor, especially during prolonged labor. Grace Burkhardt, RN, PPF Instructor and Shiatsu practitioner, developed the pressure point sequences that follow. She has used them successfully with hundreds of laboring women to ease labor pains and speed labor along. Study the pressure points and take a copy of them with you to the hospital. If you're having a home birth, have your midwife or caregiver use them on you.

Sequence #1: Sanyinjiao (Spleen #6)*

Location and Technique

- About 4 fingers lengths (3 inches) up from the inner ankle bone behind the tibia. Lie or sit down.
- Use the thumbs to press hard downward and inward toward the shin bone for 7-10 seconds, three times.

- Press during a contraction to relieve discomfort. *It may be painful.*

To Be Used For

- Any abnormalities during labor, including prolonged breech
- Difficulties during labor
- Leg cramps

Sequence #2: Taichong (Liver #3)

Location and Technique

- Over the depression between the first and second metatarsal bones. Lie or sit down.
- Use the thumbnail to press hard and inward for 7-10 seconds, three times (see Figure 11.7).

To Be Used For

- Any abnormalities during labor, including prolonged breech
- Difficulties during labor

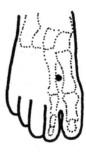

Figure 11.7 Liver #3 Pressure Point for Difficulties During Labor

---

*The number in parentheses refers to the location of that particular Shiatsu pressure point in the body.

Sequence #3: Ciliao (Urinary Bladder #32)

Location and Technique

- Press *hard* and inward with the thumbs just below the waist in the second groove of the sacrum for 5-7 seconds, three times (see Figure 11.8).

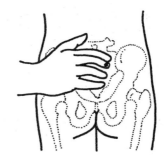

To Be Used For

- Pain and discomfort during labor, especially low back pain

Figure 11.8 Urinary Bladder #32 Pressure Point for Lessening Lower Back Pain During Labor

Sequence #4: Hoku (Large Intestine #4)

Location and Technique

- Over the dorsum of the hand, between the first and second metacarpal bone.
- Use the thumb to press *hard* against the second metacarpal bone (see Figure 11.9) for 10-15 seconds, three times.

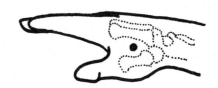

To Be Used For

- Any discomfort from the waist up

SPECIAL NOTE: Sequences 1-4 are to be used in this sequence to ensure correct results.

Figure 11.9 Large Intestine #4 Pressure Point for Lessening Pain from the Waist Up

Sequence #5: Zhiyin
(Urinary Bladder #67—"utmost female")

Location and Technique

- About one-tenth of an inch behind the lateral corner of the little toenail.
- Use the thumbnail to press down *very hard*. Do both little toes at the same time (see Figure 11.10). Press for 7-10 seconds, three times.

To Be Used For

- A difficult labor including malposition, general pain, and discomfort
- During second stage contractions, to ease delivery

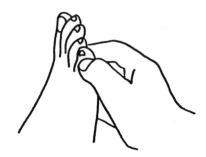

Figure 11.10 Urinary Bladder #67 Pressure Point for Second Stage Contractions to Ease Delivery

Sequence #6: Huantiao (Gall Bladder #30) and
Fengshi (Gall Bladder #31)

Location and Technique

- Press hard and inward with two thumbs on the side of the thigh (#31) and on the large indentation behind the hip (#30). (See Figure 11.11.)

To Be Used For

- Lower backache, tired legs, sciatica, or any discomfort in the lower extremities

(For a more specific discussion of Shiatsu for pregnancy, see *Shiatsu for a Healthy Pregnancy and Delivery* by Waturu Ohashi and Mary Hoover, Ballantine Books, 1984.)

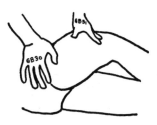

Figure 11.11 Gall Bladder #30 and #31 Pressure Points to Ease Lower Backache and Tired Legs

PERINEAL MASSAGE*

Your perineum, which is the area between your vagina and rectum, should be massaged daily beginning about the 34th week of your pregnancy. This kind of massage will prepare you for the sensations of stretching that you will feel during your baby's birth. This kind of preparation can help to reduce your need for an episiotomy. It will also reduce the risk of tearing.

Directions

1. Wash your hands. Have a mirror handy, and find a warm, private place to practice.

2. Lubricate your perineum and your thumbs with vegetable oil, cocoa butter, KY jelly, or Vitamin E oil (Vitamin E oil is the best.) You can also use your own body secretions if you wish.

3. Placing your thumbs about 1-1½ inches inside your vagina, press down and to the sides at the same time. Gently and firmly stretch the skin until you feel a slight tingling or burning sensation.

4. Continue to hold this pressure for an additional two minutes until the perineum becomes more numb and the tingling is not as distinct (see Figure 11.12).

5. Take 3-4 minutes to massage the oil into the lower half of your vagina. Avoid moving upwards toward your urethra.

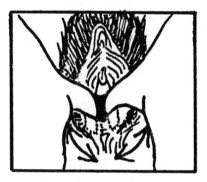

Figure 11.12 Perineal Massage

6. Pulling gently outwards or forwards, massage the lower part of your vagina with your thumbs. This massage motion helps to stretch the perineal skin, similar to the way your baby's head will stretch it during birth.

---

*Perineal Massage section adapted from "Prenatal Perineal Massage" by Elise Fleming, MA, CCE. It can be purchased in pamphlet form from ICEA, P.O. Box 20048, Minneapolis, MN 55420-0048.

Cautions and Comments

- Be sure to avoid the urethra when massaging to prevent urinary tract infections.
- Perineal massage is *not* recommended for women with an active herpes infection, since it could help the spread of lesions to other parts of the body.
- Using a mirror is helpful so you can see how your body looks.

- If you already have a healed episiotomy incision, concentrate some of the perineal massage on the area, since scar tissue is thicker and less stretchy.
- Massaging your perineum will make you more comfortable with this part of your body and is a good preparation for the upcoming birth.
- Your mate can massage your perineum if you teach him how. You will both notice how quickly this area will stretch.

SELF FACIAL MASSAGE

If you are alone and feeling a bit tense, a brief self massage can make you feel much better in a very short time. A self facial massage seems to have a profound effect on the entire body, since we carry a lot of tension in our facial muscles. You may often walk around with a scowl on your face and not even be aware of it!

Directions

1. Wash your hands. Begin the massage by taking two or three "Rock the Baby" breaths (see page 19). Place your fingers on your forehead above your eyebrows and massage across that area with moderate pressure until you come to the temples. Repeat several times.

2. Massage across your eyebrows, around the eye sockets, across closed eyes, under the eyes and up toward the temples. Massage each area until it is warm and tingly.

3. Now use your fingertips to move down each side of the nose, under your eyes and up towards the temples. Be sure to apply some pressure under each cheekbone with your thumbs.

4. Massage each side of the chin and up towards the ears. Squeeze along the chin line and massage your chin once more. Allow the jaw to open a little and be more relaxed.

5. Massage the earlobes and all along your ears, behind them and along the skull near the full length of the ears.

6. Slide your thumbs onto the skull area behind your ears and press gently, looking for tender spots. When you find a tender spot, inhale, then press on it as you exhale. Try to feel the air going to the spot you are pressing.

7. Massage along the neck looking for tender spots, then along the back and top of the head as if you were washing your hair.

8. Finally return to your forehead and stroke across it several times to finish the self massage.

Cautions and Comments

•To eliminate headaches, do a complete self massage, follow with 10 rounds of Alternate Nostril Breath (pg. 21), and finish up with 5-10 Neck Smiles (p. 72). Then, if you have a few minutes, lie down and rest for 10-15 minutes. Your headache should disappear.

•Self massage can be practiced on any part of your body—so take the time and enjoy it!

CHAPTER TWELVE
Breathing for Birth

Natural and rhythmic breathing with an inner or outer focal point is necessary for a happier and less tiring labor and delivery. You already know that learning to work with the flow of your body is an essential part of practicing the PPF program. This training is invaluable in labor because working with the natural rhythms of your laboring body will help to speed the process to its natural conclusion: the birth of your child. If you have been practicing PPF breathing during your pregnancy, you have already experienced the calming and rejuvenating effects it can have on you. During labor, controlled and rhythmic breathing serves two purposes. First, it keeps the body filled with the energy necessary for its hard work. Second, it becomes one focal point on which you may pin your awareness.

If you have been practicing PPF breathing techniques, you should have very few problems adapting to breathing for birth. PPF Breathing for Birth is very similar to the techniques taught in the Lamaze natural childbirth classes. If you are able to take a series of prepared childbirth classes with your husband or a friend, you will find this kind of training exceedingly helpful during your labor. Having a birthing assistant to monitor your breathing during labor will help you to maintain control. However, some of my students are, for a variety of reasons, unable to take any classes except for PPF. They have been able to utilize the following techniques throughout their labors. One student who had her first baby without any drugs—in two hours and twenty-five minutes—said that PPF breathing really worked!

In order for these breathing techniques to work for you, you *must* practice them daily with your birthing assistant for 10-15 minutes during the last six weeks of your pregnancy. If you are unable to take any prepared childbirth classes, explain these techniques to your birthing assistant, who can be your husband or a friend. Have your birthing assistant check to see that you are relaxed and rhythmic in your breathing, both during practice sessions and in actual labor. The more familiar you become with these breaths, the more useful and natural they will be for you during your hours of labor.

An inner or outer focal point is highly beneficial for easing you through each contraction. Some outer focal points that can be helpful include:

- the eyes of your birthing assistant, which can be very powerful
- a spot on the wall or ceiling, which can get rather dull
- a picture you really enjoy looking at
- a religious symbol, if it makes you feel protected and helped
- a Birth Mandala (see Figure 12.1), which should hold your interest

During each breathing series, you should always keep your concentration on your outer focal point.

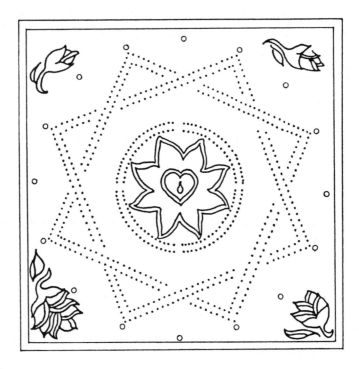

Figure 12.1 This special birth mandala can be used for outward concentration during your laboring time. Make a copy of it, color it, and pack it in your bag to take to the hospital (or use it at home).

An inner focal point may be helpful for any time during the labor when you feel yourself going inward. Mentally chanting "Om," the universal sound, is extremely powerful (it is mentally chanted: O-O-O-M-M). However, you must *not* focus on the contraction or you may lose control. Practicing your Breathing for Birth exercises with your birthing assistant will help you prepare for the hours during labor that you will share. The latest medical research indicates that women who go through labor with their husband or a friend coaching them have a more positive experience and often a shorter labor.

STAGES OF LABOR

It is wise to approach labor with the understanding that it has three basic parts. One section may go very quickly and uneventfully, while another section may prove full of complications. By mentally dividing it into sections, it will seem shorter.

The most obvious symptom of early labor is a consistent pattern of contractions. The contractions may be uneven at first, but eventually they will fall into a pattern. Contractions are usually 10-15 minutes apart at this time. Other symptoms of early labor are slight menstrual cramps, a bloody show or vaginal discharge (which is actually mucus tinged with pink rather than red), and possibly an inner feeling that the event you have been waiting for is actually beginning to happen. Many women experience the "nesting" instinct during the few days prior to the birth. You may find yourself washing floors, walls, cleaning out closets, and organizing your things in a sudden burst of energy. I remember quite well washing my kitchen floor three times during the three days prior to my first son's birth. It has never been that clean since!

Another very definite sign that labor is beginning is the breaking of your water bag, which is experienced as a warm gush of water. You may think you are urinating, but will find there is no way to control it. Placing a rolled hand towel between your legs is a good solution. You should call your doctor or midwife when these symptoms occur so that you can report on your progress. The following should be helpful to you for clarifying your understanding of labor.

Stage One: Early Labor

Characteristics

- Short, slight contractions, 10-15 minutes apart
- May not cause discomfort
- Cervix is dilated or opened 1-4 centimeters. It has to open ten centimeters (four inches) to go to Stage Two.

What to Do

- Keep moving about normally.
- Practice Salute to the Child (see page 94) to center and stay limber.
- Let your body tell you when to slow down or lie down.
- Use "Rock the Baby" or "Welcome-Farewell Breath" (p. 199), and "Early Labor Breath" (p. 199).

Stage One: Active Labor

Characteristics

- A more definite pattern of contractions, 3-5 minutes apart
- Cervix is dilated 4-8 centimeters (1½-2¼ inches)

What to Do

- Assume a comfortable position; try a variety of positions (see Chapter 13).
- Change positions frequently.
- Listen to directions from your birthing assistant on breathing and relaxing.
- Urinate every hour.
- Use "Welcome-Farewell Breath" (p. 199) and "Combined Breath" (p. 200) or any breathing pattern that is effective.
- Do a "Complete Relaxation" (p. 158) between contractions.
- Mentally talk to the baby to report on the progress the two of you are making.
- Keep your mouth relaxed throughout. Remember: "As the mouth goes, so goes the bottom."

Stage One: Transition

Characteristics

- Erratic and hard contractions, two minutes apart or less
- Feeling agitated, overwhelmed, or discouraged. These are wonderful signs, for it is almost time to push the baby out!
- Crying, feeling a sense of panic, experiencing nausea, vomiting, sweating, coldness, rectal pressure, or the shakes
- Cervix is dilated 8-10 centimeters or 3-4 inches
- The hardest but *shortest* part of labor

What to Do

- Use "Hoot and Hout Breath" (p. 201) and "Blowing Breath" (p. 202).
- Listen to your birthing assistant. Concentrate on your outer or inner focus to maintain control.
- *Do not push* even if you have the urges: pant or blow instead.
- Mentally keep telling yourself (and the baby, too) that this difficult stage will be over very shortly.
- Try to be in the "here and now" by handling one contraction at a time. Do not anticipate the next one.

Stage Two: Your Baby's Birth

Characteristics

- Strong contractions, further apart and much less intense
- A very strong urge to push, as you do when you have to move your bowels
- A burning sensation on the pelvic floor or a feeling of a giant bowel movement

What to Do

- Push when told, using "Pushing Breath" (p. 203).
- Relax your mouth and pelvic floor muscles.
- Relax completely between pushes.
- Pant or blow if you are told *not* to push.
- Use an upright sitting or squatting position with support for the best results.
- Watch your baby being born!

Stage Three: Birth of the Placenta

Characteristics

- Continuing uterine contractions, which will slowly come to a stop
- If you have had an episiotomy, your doctor or midwife will be suturing it at this time. You will receive local anesthesia for this procedure.

What to Do

- Using "Pushing Breath" (p. 203), push the placenta out.
- Use any breathing technique you want during subsiding contractions.

The state of consciousness right after the baby is born has been described by many women as "a super wonderful high." The body and the mind generate vast amounts of energy for your baby to arrive. Enjoy this heightened consciousness and excitement if it comes. If you have received drugs during your labor and delivery, you will probably still feel this "baby high."

You will have to wait and see if any drugs will be necessary for your birth experience. Place your trust and faith in your doctor or midwife to guide you in this area.

If you approach labor as a positive experience for which you are well prepared and energized, you will be able to face all the challenges that come along. Labor means hard, long, sweaty, intense work. You are going to be hot; you are going to be tired; you may wonder if you will run out of energy. Do not go into labor with any preconceived notions such as "I will not take any medication," or "I know this labor is going to last forever," or "I know this is going to be as easy as can be." Accept your laboring experience, work with it by using your breathing and having faith in your own inner strength.

BIRTH ASSISTANT'S CHECKLIST

During Pre- or Early Labor: (1-3 cms.):

1. Encourage the laboring woman to sleep or at least conserve her energy.

2. Suggest that she take a warm bath or shower if her membranes have not broken. Help her to get in and out of the bath.

3. Unless she is nauseous, suggest that she drink natural fruit juice, red raspberry leaf tea with honey, or frozen orange juice concentrate with honey and a little water. These fluids will provide quick energy. Birthing assistants should remember to eat during labor.

4. Time her contractions when they begin. Note the interval between contractions and the length of each contraction. Also note when her membranes rupture and whether she has a "bloody show."

5. Before leaving for the hospital or place of birth, pack some food for the hours of labor. Try to bring foods with mild odors so as not to distract the laboring woman.

6. The laboring woman should practice "Rock the Baby" Breath (see page 19).

During Mid-Labor: (3-7 cms.):

1. When you arrive at the hospital try to sign in quickly. Have your insurance cards and numbers handy so forms can be completed easily.

2. When assisting the laboring woman through her contractions— *be positive. Don't criticize* or dwell on the negative. Keep your "Breathing for Birth" pamphlet handy so that you can check on which breaths to use and when.

3. Make sure the laboring woman takes two "Rock the Baby" or "Welcome-Farewell" (see page 199) breaths at the beginning and end of each contraction.

4. Breathe with her when the going gets rough. This will help her to keep a slow rhythm. She may want to use your eyes as a focal point. If she seems to stray, tell her: "Open your eyes and look at me—I'll breathe with you."

5. Wipe her face with a cool cloth; massage her back or legs between contractions; massage the abdomen very lightly; hold her hand. Try to be as physical as possible—as far as she allows. If the labor slows down or stops, couples are encouraged to kiss passionately. Gentle nipple stimulation by the birthing assistant, if this is acceptable to the couple, will often get the labor going again *without the use of drugs.*

6. *Remind the laboring woman to keep her mouth loose between contractions.* This is helpful for relaxing the birth canal area.

7. Remind the laboring woman to empty her bladder every hour. Walking is very helpful in speeding up labor. Be sure to stay near her at all times.

8. Keep up with her moods. Talk if she wants to, play cards, or encourage her to doze between contractions. If she is on a fetal monitor, make her aware of any upcoming contractions so she isn't taken by surprise.

9. If medication is offered, encourage her to wait another few minutes before taking any. Demerol, which is often administered during labor, causes grogginess and an inability to breathe through contractions.

During Transition: (7-10 cms.):

1. Try hard to get her to relax.

2. Don't ask any questions that require more than a "yes" or "no" answer.

3. Wipe her face if she seems warm. Offer her ice chips or lollipops between contractions if the doctor or midwife approves.

4. Spread chapstick on her lips when her mouth feels dry.

5. The laboring woman may get very crabby, nasty, tired, etc. Don't react to her moods. Instead *try to remain positive.*

6. If she feels sick and wants to throw up, get her a basin and encourage her to do so. She will feel better afterwards.

7. When she begins to make grunting or "pushing" sounds, contact her doctor or midwife immediately. Keep breath-

ing with her through the end of transition and until she is fully dilated.

8. Have her use Hoot-Hout Breathing or Blowing Breath.

During Pushing:

1. Change into appropriate hospital gear for delivery. Do so quickly so as not to be away from the laboring woman for too long.

2. You may have to move into the delivery room or else remain in the birthing room, depending upon the circumstances of the birth.

3. Remind the laboring woman to relax her pelvic floor muscles during pushing. Hold her up if she needs support during the peak of each contraction. Encourage her to take a deep breath and push with a controlled exhalation. She should push four times during each contraction.

4. Encourage her after each push by saying: "The baby is almost here," "One more good push will do it," etc.

5. If an emergency occurs in the delivery room and you're asked to leave, don't argue. But this isn't a usual occurrence.

6. Finally, after all those long hours of hard work, the baby that you have waited so long for arrives. Congratulations!

CHECKLIST FOR LABOR

____ two small cosmetic or artist's sponges (natural ones are best) to use for moistening the laboring woman's mouth, putting water on her face

____ wide-mouth thermos bottle for holding ice chips

____ toilet bag containing toothbrush, soap, washcloth, deodorant, make-up, etc.

____ hairbrush, comb, ribbons (for long hair)

____ talcum powder (unscented or lightly scented) and oil or lotion for massage

____ small aerosol or garden spray can to be filled with cold water for refreshing the woman's face

____ eau de cologne (not musky—plain bath cologne is best)

____ vitamin E oil (wheat germ oil) for massaging the birth canal area in preparation for delivery

____ Vaseline, chapstick or lip gloss for dry lips

____ picnic freezer bag or ice bag to be used as a cold compress

____ hot water bottle to be used as a warm compress

____ neck cushion or pillow to support the woman's head comfortably forward

____ inflatable beach ball for knees or small of the back

____ warm socks

____ food for the birthing assistant during labor and perhaps for the new mother after the baby is born

____ notebook and a pen for a labor log

____ change for phone calls, list of telephone numbers of close friends and relatives

____ nursing nightgowns, bras, slippers, panties

____ baby clothes and birth announcements to be written out

____ ear plugs, in case the laboring woman finds the surrounding noises distracting

____ watch, camera, sour candy, lollipops

BREATHS FOR LABOR AND BIRTH

Welcome-Farewell Breath
("Rock the Baby" Breath)

Benefits

- Mentally signals the beginning and end of each contraction
- Keeps the body relaxed and well supplied with oxygen

Directions

1. Keeping the facial and tummy muscles relaxed, inhale through the nose, rocking the baby forward.

2. Exhale slowly either through your nose or through a loosely opened mouth. Repeat.

Cautions and Comments

- You should be *very* familiar with this breath, having used it all through pregnancy!
- Treat each contraction as a unique experience or wave. Welcome it with a breath, breathe through it, and then say goodbye to it with a breath. Repeat.
- Keep these breaths slow, rhythmic, and even.

Early Labor Breath

Benefits

- Keeps the uterus and your body well supplied with oxygen
- Focuses your attention away from the contraction, thereby lessening your perception of pain

Directions

1. As the contraction begins, take one or two Welcome-Farewell Breaths (see page 199). Slowly inhale through your nose, sending the air to your chest area. Your tummy will move out, but keep your awareness on the chest area expanding forward with each inhalation.

2. As you inhale, think: "In, two, three, four." As you exhale, think: "Out, two, three, four."

3. Keep your breathing even and your focus on counting each breath, as well as on your outside focal point.

4. You should take 6-10 Early Labor Breaths during each 60-second contraction.

5. Always keep your mind on your breathing and counting.

6. When the contraction is ending, do one or two Welcome-Farewell Breaths (see page 199) and resume normal breathing until the next contraction begins.

Cautions and Comments

- Develop a comfortable inhalation and exhalation count.
- Keep your inhalations and exhalations smooth, even, and rhythmic.
- Try to use your nose for inhaling and exhaling.

Combined Breath (For Mid-Labor)

Benefits

- Increases the need for concentration by changing the rate of the breath, thereby lessening the perception of pain
- Keeps the diaphragm up and away from the uterus during the peak of the contraction
- Keeps the body and the baby well supplied with energy

Directions

1. When the contraction begins, take one or two Welcome-Farewell breaths (see page 199). Use Early Labor breath (see page 199) until the contraction begins to peak and you need to switch to Mouth-Centered Breathing.

2. Mouth-Centered Breathing is a shallow in-out mouth breath with an increased rate. Use the sounds "hoot" and "hout" as a pattern on which you can concentrate. Make sure you say each sound for at least one second. Also be sure that you cross your T's at the end of each sound to keep your mouth moist.

3. When the contraction has peaked and begins to subside, return to Early Labor breath (see page 199) and finish the contraction with one or two Welcome-Farewell Breaths (see page 199).

Cautions and Comments

- This pattern will work well during the middle stages of labor when the cervix is opening from approximately 3-7 centimeters ($1^1/_2$-$2^3/_4$ inches).
- You must keep your mouth open and relaxed during Mouth-Centered Breathing.
- You may want to invent your own patterns for using the Early Labor breath. You may want to inhale/exhale for five, then reduce it the next time to four, then three, and so on.
- Using "hoot" and "hout" while keeping your tummy muscles relaxed will eliminate the need to think about inhaling and exhaling. The air will simply move in and out without your thinking about it.

Hoot and Hout Breath

Benefits

- Increased mental concentration for switching patterns keeps your awareness away from the forceful contractions
- Keeps the diaphragm up and away from the contracting uterus, thereby facilitating your labor
- Keeps your mind occupied at a time when you may be ready to give up and go home

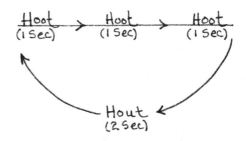

Figure 12.2 Smile Pattern for "Hoot and Hout" Breathing

Directions

1. Begin your contraction with one or two Welcome-Farewell breaths (see page 199).

2. Have your birth assistant stand in front of you and mark off the seconds with his or her hand in a Smile Pattern (see Figure 12.2). You should take five seconds to say the Hoot and Hout sounds: three seconds for the Hoot sound and two seconds for the Hout sound.

3. As the contraction heightens (which will be very quickly), begin to say Hoot-Hoot-Hoot-Hout in a very rhythmic way as you do Mouth-Centered Breathing. Continue to follow your birth assistant's hand pattern with your eyes as you breathe.

4. Use Hoot and Hout Breathing through the entire contraction and finish with one or two Welcome-Farewell breaths (see page 199).

Variations

To make the concentration more complicated, vary this breath by using the following patterns:

> Hoot-Hoot-Hoot-Hout
> Hoot-Hoot-Hout
> Hoot-Hout
> Hoot

or

> Hout
> Hoot-Hout
> Hoot-Hoot-Hout
> Hoot-Hoot-Hoot-Hout

or

> 4 Hoots + 1 Hout
> 6 Hoots + 1 Hout
> 2 Hoots + 1 Hout, etc.

or invent your own patterns.

Cautions and Comments

- Contractions during transition will last anywhere from 60-90 seconds with very little time between. They seem to tumble upon each other.
- Watching the movement of your birth assistant's hand contributes to the calming effect of this breath. It seems to partially hypnotize you when you need it the most.
- The breathing may make your mouth dry. Making the "t" sound will help. You may want to have an ice chip between contractions.
- Your husband or birth assistant should indicate which beat you should be on. Total concentration on this breath is necessary in order to keep control.
- The transition period of labor completes the opening of the cervix and is the most intense section of labor for most women. At this point you may feel as if you want to throw in the towel and go home. You may feel nauseated, very cold or very hot, very emotional or very tired. You may not want your husband near you or touching you. You may find that you are in another state of consciousness during transition. You are—so experience it, for your baby will soon be born.

Blowing Breath

Benefits

- Redirects and diminishes the pushing urge until the proper time
- Lets out a variety of tensions and emotions

Directions

1. During a contraction while you are using the Hoot-Hout breath, you may want to bear down and push. This is inadvisable until the cervix is fully dilated. Instead, you can puff your cheeks out and blow out hard as if you are blowing out several candles on a cake.
2. The breathing pattern would look like this: Welcome-Farewell → Hoot-Hout (repeated) → Blowing Breath → Hoot-Hout (repeated) → Welcome-Farewell.
3. Puff your cheeks and blow in short bursts. Repeat all during the urge to push.

Cautions and Comments

- Pushing during transition may tear your cervix and make the labor last longer.
- Blowing should be used only when you have the urge to push and should not. Panting may be substituted for blowing if you are more comfortable with it. You can pant by keeping your mouth slightly open and inhaling and exhaling quickly.

Pushing Breath

Benefits

- Enables the body to bear down and push the baby through the birth canal and into this life
- Enables you to adequately utilize the oxygen in your system at the moment

Directions

1. As the contraction begins, in a relaxation position, take 1-2 Welcome-Farewell breaths (see page 199). Take a deep breath and then bear down as you control your exhalation through an opened mouth. When you run out of air, take another deep breath and bear down, exhaling through your mouth as you push. Making sounds seems to help many women to push.

2. Repeat this about four times during the contraction.

3. As the contraction begins to subside, return to a relaxation position; finish off with 1-2 Welcome-Farewell breaths (see page 199).

4. Relax and breathe normally until the next contraction begins.

Cautions and Comments

- You need to push down, up, and out, for that is the route your baby will take. Use your full lungs and abdominal muscles to push down.
- You have to think "down" as you push. Do not push in your face or you will burst blood vessels.
- You do not have to push with every contraction.
- You may be quite noisy when you push. This is fine.
- Push through your birth canal, not your anus. Pushing in the anal area causes postpartum hemorrhoids.
- You may hear the doctor, midwife, or nurses telling you to blow during the pushing stage, for they do not want your baby to be born too quickly. Use Blowing Breath (see page 202) during these sections of the pushing phase.
- You push with the same vaginal muscles you used in "Baby Breath" (p. 23).
- You have to push during contractions to deliver the placenta out as well.
- Women having a second or third child will have afterbirth uterine contractions through which they will have to breathe for comfort.
- The baby will move down with each push and then slip back. At times it may seem frustrating. Finally, the baby's head will leave the birth canal. Birth of the entire baby will follow very soon.
- The latest research indicates that holding your breath while pushing goes against the body's natural desire to push. By taking a deep breath, bearing down *as you control the exhalation*, you will gently ease your baby down and out and help prevent your perineum from tearing.
- Making vocal sounds seems to help many women with the pushing process. It also releases tensions.

CHAPTER THIRTEEN

Advantageous Positions for Labor and Birth

You are not sick when you are in labor! You do not have to retire to your bed but are free to walk around, and move in and out of several positions during some of the time. Your freedom of movement is based to a great extent on where you choose to give birth. If you are having a home birth, you will obviously be able to move about as you and the circumstances permit. If you have a hospital birth, you may find that you have to stay in bed for the last part of the labor, especially if you have a birth monitor on your abdomen recording information about your baby. In either case, it is wise to become familiar with as many of the following laboring and birthing positions as you can. Many women have found that shifting out of an ineffectual position into a new one often speeds the progress of the labor and birth.

Laboring positions which tilt the torso forward utilize the force of gravity to help the laboring, pushing and birth process along. If you are in a conventional hospital setting, you may not be able to utilize some of the suggested pushing positions. If that is the case, follow the directions that you received in your prenatal education classes or from the hospital staff. If you are having a home birth with a midwife, you should become totally familiar with the pushing positions which are included here by practicing them during the last six weeks of your pregnancy. Shifting into a variety of positions makes labor *seem* shorter. Try practicing your Breathing for Birth breaths in all of these laboring positions so you can learn which positions are the most comfortable. Many of the squatting and kneeling positions help to keep the pelvic and birth canal areas of your body in good tone.

HELPFUL POSITIONS FOR THE EARLY AND MID FIRST STAGE OF LABOR

1. Walking around and stopping for contractions

2. Lying down for resting or sleeping; use the side-lying position

3. Sitting and leaning on the back of a chair (see Figure 13.1). Put a pillow on the top of the chair for comfort.

4. Sitting in the Zen Sitting position (see page 102) with the knees open while resting on a chair (see Figure 13.2).

5. Standing and leaning against the wall during contractions. Cradle your arms against the wall and rest your head on them.

6. Squatting on heels or toes while holding onto a chair for support.

7. Cross-legged sitting position (p. 122).

8. Holding your birthing assistant for comfort and leaning forward (see Figure 13.3).

9. Any other positions that you find comfortable.

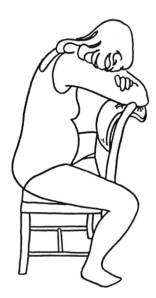

Figure 13.1   Sitting and Leaning on the Back of a Chair

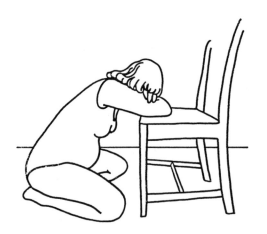

Figure 13.2   Zen Sitting Position with the Knees Open Resting on a Chair

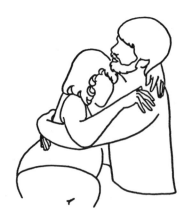

Figure 13.3   Holding Onto Your Birth Assistant for Support

ADVANTAGEOUS POSITIONS FOR LATE FIRST STAGE OF LABOR (TRANSITION)

1. Kneeling onto a chair with the knees separated and head up.

2. One leg bent and flat; the other leg in a kneeling position. Arms should rest on a chair. Shift legs between contractions (see Figure 13.4).

3. The Rainbow position with the back rounded a bit (see Figure 7.59). Place your arms on a chair in this position if they get tired.

4. Sitting and leaning forward while holding onto your birth assistant (see Figure 13.5).

5. A semi-sitting, semi-reclining position with several pillows under your back. Your knees can be bent or you can have the legs flat (this is the best position in bed). See Figure 8.1.

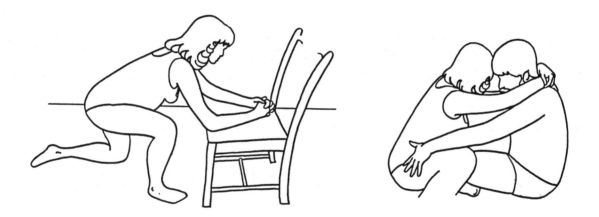

Figure 13.4 One Leg Kneeling, the Other Flat, and Arms on a Chair   **Figure 13.5** Your Labor Assistant Breathing with You During a Contraction

USEFUL POSITIONS FOR THE SECOND STAGE OF LABOR (PUSHING)

1. Squatting on toes or flat feet while bearing down holding onto a chair (see Figure 13.6). You can lean your back against the wall in this position as well.

2. Kneeling and leaning forward onto a chair for pushing (see Figure 13.2).

3. The Rainbow Position (see Figure 7.59).

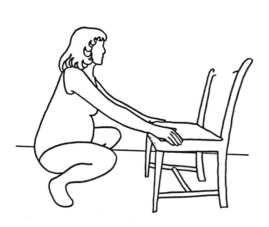

Figure 13.6   Squatting on Toes Near a Chair   **Figure 13.7**   Your Birth Assistant Holding
                                                                       You in a Squatting Position

4. Pushing in a semi-sitting reclining position with the legs open and knees bent.
    Have a wedge or some pillows behind you to retain this position. Place your hands
    underneath your knees, or place bent legs on bars on each side of the bed, or up in
    stirrups during the contraction to facilitate pushing.

5. One leg kneeling, other leg flat, arms resting on a chair.

6. Have your birthing assistant assist you by holding you underneath the arms in a
    squatting position. She or he can lean against a wall in this position (see Figure
    13.7).

These positions are only suggestions to which you can add your own. You will find
that you change positions often during labor, so being familiar with a variety of movements can be helpful, especially during long labors. If you are in bed during labor, you
can still go into some of the kneeling positions by turning sideways and using the bars
on the sides of the bed for support. *Do not use a flat back reclining position for labor and birth
because it cuts down on circulation and forces your body to work against gravity.*

Introduce these different positions to your mate or birthing assistant before you go
into labor. You may forget many of these movements, but hopefully your birthing
assistant will remember. Changing positions often will give you something else to
think about during labor and delivery. A variety of laboring and birthing positions,
controlled breathing and inner faith will all help contribute to a more positive birth
experience.

CHAPTER FOURTEEN
A Primer for the Nursing Mother

Breastfeeding is the natural completion of the physical union and compatibility that you have been experiencing throughout your pregnancy. It is merely a voluntary continuation of an involuntary process.

The decision to breastfeed or bottlefeed your baby is a very personal one and should be discussed with your mate. It is one of the first decisions you will make in your roles as new parents. By doing some reading, and talking to other women who have successfully nursed their babies, you will gather much information on which to base your decision. It is advisable to attend a local meeting of La Leche League, which is a nonprofit organization concerned with teaching women how to successfully breastfeed their babies. Your doctor or midwife will probably have the name of your local group leader.

Medical research in this area has indicated that nursing your baby can be highly beneficial for the baby's growth and development, as well as for your own body. Some of the most important benefits of nursing are:

1. *Nutrition*. Your breast milk is perfect for fulfilling your baby's nutritional needs. It is freshly made and can be rapidly and easily digested by your baby.

2. *Health*. Immunities to certain diseases for the first two years of the baby's life are contained in colostrum, which is produced during pregnancy and is consumed by the baby during the first few days of breastfeeding.

3. *Availability*. Breast milk is available immediately, at the right temperature, and in the right quantity wherever you go.

4. *Digestion*. The stools of breastfed babies are loose, mustard-colored, and have a mild odor. Constipation is rarely a problem.

5. *Economy*. Breast milk is economical and a great natural resource. You have only to add one additional serving of calcium foods and 500 calories daily to your well-balanced diet to produce more than enough milk for your baby.

6. *Relaxation*. The time that you and your baby spend together during each feeding forces you to sit down, put your feet up, breathe deeply, and relax for good milk letdown and flow. This shared experience several times a day fosters a close physical and emotional relationship that can be enjoyed by both mother and baby.

If you have been persuaded to strongly consider nursing your baby, you should begin actively preparing both mentally and physically. Mental attitude regarding your breasts and the way you will be using them as a nursing mother has a very important bearing on your breastfeeding experience. The duality of the female body is most evident during pregnancy, birth, and lactation; during these times the primarily sexual parts of the body will be used for very different purposes.

By accepting the very beautiful and utilitarian duality of your body, you may better adjust to the use of the breasts for nourishment of your child as well as for the sexual stimulation of your body during lovemaking. Since you cannot entirely separate these two physical functions, you may feel somewhat sexually stimulated while you are doing nipple preparation. Accept these pleasurable feelings and enjoy them. You may feel sexual sensations while you are nursing your baby; these are a perfectly normal and natural part of a very close physical union or bond.

PRENATAL NIPPLE PREPARATION

Nipple preparation, especially for fair-haired women, can help to minimize sore nipples once the baby begins to nurse. Nipple preparation cannot always eliminate the effects of engorgement, constant poor positioning of the baby at the breast, and other complications. However, well-prepared, healthy skin will be more resistant to irritation and will heal more quickly if it does become damaged. Therefore, it is wise to take the precaution of doing some form of prenatal nipple preparation.

During pregnancy, hormones act on the breast to prepare it for breastfeeding. In order to accommodate internal breast development, the skin stretches and becomes more pliable. The nipple and areola (brown part of the nipple) enlarge and are protected by increased pigmentation. The Montgomery glands located on the areola have a pimply appearance and secrete an oily substance that serves as lubricant and protective agent for the nipple. The keratin, or dead skin layer, of your skin protects you against infection. You want to work with the natural processes already in progress inside your pregnant body in order to derive the full benefit from nipple preparation. You are encouraged to do the following:

Do's

1. *Do* expose your breasts to air and sunlight during the last three months of pregnancy. You should sunbathe topless *no more* than twenty minutes because sensitive skin burns very easily. If you wear a nursing bra, wear it with the flaps down, or go braless for part of the day.

2. *Do* massage your breasts when showering but *do not* wash the nipples with soap. This will remove the protective layers that your skin is naturally providing.

3. *Do* enjoy breast stimulation during sexual activity.

Don'ts

1. *Do not* use soap or any drying agent on the nipples.

2. *Do not* use plastic liners in your breast pads.

3. *Do not* use artificial lubricants unless you need them.

4. *Do not* use any lubricant that does not allow your skin to breathe or must be washed off.

5. *Do not* rub your nipples with a towel or washcloth, for that will only remove the layer of keratin.

6. *Do not* wear tight bras and other restrictive clothing, since localized pressure on breast tissue can cause discomfort and result in plugged milk ducts.

7. *Do not* use a nipple shield during breastfeeding, for it interferes with the proper milking of the breast and may lead to poor weight gain for your baby.

CORRECT BABY POSITIONING TO ELIMINATE SORE NIPPLES

When learning to breastfeed your baby, you may experience very sore nipples *if* your baby is positioned incorrectly. Try to follow these simple rules for correct baby positioning to ensure that breastfeeding is a rewarding experience.

1. Wash your hands.

2. Hold your baby in the crook of your arm, with your hand on your baby's buttocks or upper thigh.

3. Hold your breast by placing four fingers beneath it and your thumb on top, making sure that your hand is not on the areola. *Do not* tilt the nipple up because this will incorrectly position your nipple in the baby's mouth and cause sore nipples.

4. Bring your baby to the breast, *not your breast to the baby*. Point the nipple down and lightly tickle the baby's lower lip. Your baby should open his or her mouth widely as if taking a yawn.

5. Pull your baby close and put the child *on the breast*, not just on the nipple. Your baby's *hips, stomach, and head should face your body at the level of the breast*. You may need pillows and the arm of your rocking chair for support and comfort.

6. If you had a c/section, place pillows beneath your abdomen. Have your baby on its side facing you. Roll toward the baby, placing the entire breast in baby's mouth. You can use a bath pan at the foot of the bed to support your legs and prevent slipping down in bed. Don't lean over to nurse in bed, for that will cause a sore back.

EQUIPMENT FOR BREASTFEEDING

One piece of equipment that will enhance your nursing experience is a rocking chair. Your baby has been rocked throughout its 9-month stay inside your body, and the movement of a rocking chair can be very relaxing for both of you. The rocking chair that you choose should have a high enough back to support your head, and should have arms that will maximize comfort when holding the baby (see Figure 14.1). Take your time as you shop. Sit in a number of chairs until you find one that fits your body size

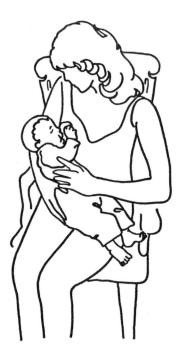

Figure 14.1   Using a Rocking Chair
While Nursing the Baby

and shape. A footstool or hassock is also a good idea so that you can put up your feet as you nurse. This aids your blood circulation while adding to your comfort and relaxation.

Another necessity for breastfeeding is a breast pump, which you can use to empty your breasts when they are too full or to pump out milk for future use. There are new pumps on the market that come with detachable bottles for easy and quick milk collection. Your mate can feed your baby after you pump your breasts. Breast milk may be frozen for up to two weeks in the refrigerator freezer and in a deep freeze for six months to two years. Thaw in warm water but *don't* microwave it, for it can burn your baby's lips and mouth.

The Happy Family Breast Milking and Feeding Unit is available through PPF. See the Appendix for ordering instructions.

MISCONCEPTIONS ABOUT NURSING

Many women believe they will be continuously tied to the baby if they breastfeed. However, many breastfed babies will take a bottle of previously pumped breast milk or formula when their mother is not available. There are many working women who nurse their babies only in the morning and evening and give the baby formula during the day. The frequency of nursing is something that you and your baby can work out.

If you are separated from your baby and your breasts become full, you can easily hand-express the extra milk in the nearest bathroom sink. If you have difficulty hand-expressing, you can carry your breast pump with you to eliminate the extra milk.

Another misconception is that you will not be able to make nutritious milk in adequate supply for your baby. You will be able to make enough nutritionally-balanced milk for your baby to grow and develop as long as you include 500 extra calories a day plus one extra serving of calcium-rich foods in your postpartum diet, chosen wisely from the four basic food groups. Your body will do the rest. Your natural "milk machine" will continue to supply your baby for as long as you like.

Small-breasted women often question their ability to produce adequate supplies of milk. The size of the breast has very little to do with its ability to produce enough milk. Much of a woman's milk supply is stored in the back of her breasts. As the baby sucks out the front milk, the stored milk is drawn forward and consumed.

Before the invention of formula, women had little choice about breastfeeding their babies. It was simply an accepted part of the motherhood role. Learning about nursing and experiencing it even for a short time will deepen your understanding of how the female body functions. If you find that nursing is not right for you, you can easily put your baby on formula. Since you do have both options open to you, the PPF approach would be the natural way first.

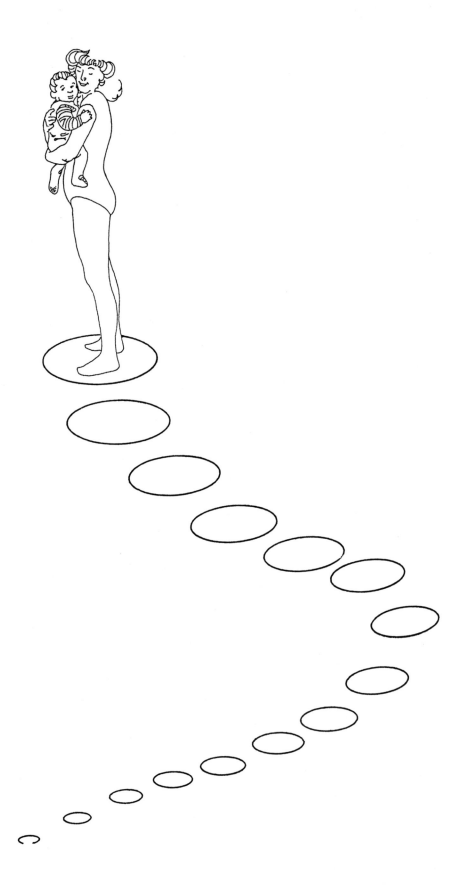

CHAPTER FIFTEEN

Four Personal Birth Stories

Reading about someone else's birth experience can be most helpful in preparing you for your own. Often, a personal word or comment can give you more insight into childbirth than all the books that have been written on the subject. The following four stories reflect a variety of options that are available to you at the present time.

HOME BIRTH

Eileen and Mark chose to have their first child, Sara Anne, born December 6, 1985, at home. She was born with only one midwife attending.

Eileen tells their story: "When we became pregnant with our first child, we planned a home birth with our friend and nurse-midwife, Marge. Along with good nutrition and exercise, I focused much of my energy on forming and reaffirming a positive attitude toward birth for myself. The PPF Teacher Training Workshop that I attended toward the end of my pregnancy was very helpful in this respect. As with any first-time mother, I had all the 'normal' fears that only the actual birth could erase.

"One of the issues that I struggled with was that of control. As a midwife myself, I know that one must 'surrender' to the strength and power of the body in labor. My greatest fear was that I would be unable to give up control when labor began. I used the PPF relaxation/visualization techniques to reaffirm my trust in my ability to give birth.

"When my membranes ruptured just a few days after my due date, I lay in bed holding my husband's hand, feeling both excited and surprised by the strength of my first contractions. It was nice to know that we were where we planned to be for this birth. Mark stayed home from work to finish some last minute chores and to keep me company.

"The contractions became irregular and remained that way until late in the evening, despite all the 'tricks of the trade.' By bedtime, they had almost disappeared and I had come to terms with the possibility of a radically different type of birth than the one we had originally planned; i.e., having to go to the hospital. Such despair!!!

"After a much needed cry on Mark's shoulder, a visualization, a glass of wine, and Marge's constant assurance that I would go into labor soon, I went to bed and immediately began active labor. The contractions quickly went from fifteen, to five, to two minutes apart. There was no question as to who was in control now—Mother Nature was !!

"With each contraction becoming stronger than the last, it took great concentration to get through each one. After trying to get comfortable in several positions, I found leaning against Mark in bed to be the most tolerable. After two hours of contractions Mark awakened Marge, who had stayed with us all day. Her initial exam showed that I was seven centimeters dilated. Mark then called our birth assistants, Lori and Maggie, who also happened to be our friends.

"Maggie had agreed to take photos for us and found herself helping to rub my legs with each contraction. That was a great help. Marge and Lori talked to me in very positive terms, describing what my body was doing: 'Your cervix is stretching around the baby's head' or 'Imagine how good it will feel to hold your baby in your arms.' These were the very words that I had 'rehearsed' so many times during visualizations. This really helped me to focus positively on the pain. My husband Mark was wonderful. He was calm and kept reassuring me that I could do it, especially when transition dragged on. The baby was in a posterior position, with the back of her head resting on my spine. Turning onto my left side helped the baby to move down. After another hour, I began pushing spontaneously. Again progress was slow because the baby had not yet rotated to an anterior position. Marge suggested many position changes to help the baby to turn.

"After an hour and a half, I finally brought the baby down low enough to rotate into the right birthing position. Pushing with all my strength on my right side was very effective. Soon I felt an incredible stretching feeling as my baby's head was born. I was extremely noisy as I pushed. That felt really good.

"Sara was born with the next push at 8:01 A.M., weighing eight pounds, twelve ounces. It was such a marvelous feeling to look down at this precious gift, so perfectly formed. It was such an incredible feeling to hold her at last and share hugs and kisses all around. Since I didn't need stitches, I took a shower while Mark and Sara got acquainted. We made lots of phone calls to announce Sara's arrival. Then we celebrated her birth with a wonderful champagne and omelette breakfast."

HOSPITAL BIRTH WITH COMPLICATIONS

Jacquie, an R.N., a PPF teacher and a Positive Parenting Fitness Master Teacher, tells about Seth's birth: "My husband Keith and I chose to travel to Hartford, over an hour away, for the birth of our second child. One of a group of four nurse-midwives would be assisting us. They were backed up by an excellent group of obstetricians.

"I'd had a great deal of Braxton-Hicks contractions with this pregnancy. The contractions gradually became more regular as my pregnancy progressed. Because of the distance, and the quick labor and delivery of my first child, we had planned to start for Hartford at the onset of labor. Even if we arrived in Hartford early in labor, we planned to do some Christmas shopping.

"On Sunday, December 9th, the contractions were mild, seven minutes apart and very consistent. We went to a local tree farm that afternoon for our Christmas tree. By Sunday night the contractions were regular, even through the activity of trimming the tree. On Monday morning I called the midwife. She made an appointment for me at 11:30 A.M. that day for a check, provided I didn't go into active labor, in which case I would go right in. I saw the midwife and she was a little concerned that fetal activity had slowed down. She wanted a strip on the fetal monitor. I was admitted for what was to be forty-five minutes to an hour. The monitor showed my baby's heart rate to be a little slow, and there was a slight dip after each contraction. This, combined with the decreased activity, concerned her. Thus she contacted the obstetrician for a consultation.

"The obstetrician, who seemed compassionate and sincere, informed me that in 'his' opinion the baby was fine, but he recommended that my water be broken. This procedure, he assured me, would almost surely induce labor. Then an internal monitor could be attached to my baby's head so he could get a more accurate reading of what was happening. In that way, he could have more control over my labor, rather than send me home. He made the procedure sound very simple. Even my husband was in favor of it.

"After hearing my choices, however, I flatly refused all these intervening procedures. I sensed that my baby was fine and would be born in his own time.

"My husband and I had decided to stay in the hospital overnight awaiting the onset of labor. But then I was told, 'Just in case you go into labor, we have to put you on a liquid diet.' I had gotten to the hospital at 11:30 A.M. It was now 4:00 P.M. I didn't eat any lunch or dinner and I was famished. The hospital staff recommended an I.V. (intravenous feeding via a needle in your arm). But instead, we decided to go to a hotel in Hartford.

"We went out to a nice restaurant and had a big meal. We were disappointed when labor did not start that night. The next day, we went Christmas shopping. Late in the afternoon, we drove home.

"The next morning, at 5:30 A.M., I woke up with mild menstrual-type contractions. I had the feeling that this was it but I wanted to be sure this time. Keith was outside installing paneling in his van. He didn't plan on going into work not until after the baby was born. We knew with all the false labor that real labor was imminent. By 6:30 A.M., I knew these contractions were very regular and different from the Braxton-Hicks contractions I had been feeling previously.

"I got up and showered. By this time Keith had come in and he was all excited. I called the midwife, and by 7:30 A.M. we were on our way toward Hartford again.

"I dreaded the ride because it would be long and I would not be able to move around very much. Once in the car, I began Welcome-Farewell breaths and felt quite comfortable. But about two-thirds of the way to Hartford, this breathing was no longer effective. I began Early Labor Breathing—inhaling for four and exhaling for four with great relief. I must admit I was amazed at what a difference the breathing made. To complicate the ride I had a full bladder and was in the middle of rush-hour traffic. But inhaling and exhaling at a slow and easy pace kept me comfortable. We arrived at the hospital at about 8:30 A.M. When I was finally checked, I was six centimeters dilated.

"The contractions were five minutes apart. Labor progressed gradually, as my contractions became stronger and closer. By 10:00 A.M. my contractions were very strong. I began the pattern of Hoot-Hoot-Hoot-Hout as Keith moved his hand through the air. He was a little concerned that it might be too early, but the mid-labor breath was no longer effective.

"I had back labor, so Keith massaged my back and applied counter pressure. We listened to soothing music throughout the labor. Contractions became even stronger and closer. I got up to go to the bathroom and as I walked back to bed, a contraction began. It caught me off guard and I did not begin the breath. It was almost unbearable. It made me realize how effective the breathing was. By 10:30 A.M. the Hoot-Hoot-Hoot-Hout became very loud and came from deep within me. But it felt so good to groan it out. I kept thinking, 'They must be able to hear me all the way down the hall.' But that did not quiet me down!

"By 10:40 A.M., I did not think I could take it much longer. My midwife checked me and said I was ready to push. Using controlled exhalation and plenty of noise, I began pushing. It was very effective. Just three feet from the foot of the bed was a wall mirror. It went from the floor to the ceiling and was wider than the bed. I could see the baby's head coming out. Seeing it seemed to give me renewed strength and, with a few more pushes, Seth was born. My beautiful baby boy weighed eight pounds, ten ounces.

"He was placed on my tummy and in a few minutes I was able to nurse him. He did not nurse as readily as my daughter had, but after a little coaching, he did fine.

"My placenta was delivered and it appeared to be intact. The nurse began massaging my fundus (the top of my uterus). But I was passing large clots and a large amount of blood. My fundus was boggy and wasn't contracting. Medication was administered with no effect. After consulting with the obstetrician, the midwife started a Pitocin drip IV with the hope that this procedure would stop the bleeding. Unfortunately, the bleeding and clots continued.

"By 4:00 P.M. I saw the physician and he informed me that a D&C (dilation of the cervix and curettage or scraping of the uterus) was in order. Being a nurse myself, I knew it was coming!

"Suddenly, I recalled a woman I knew who had hemorrhaged profusely following the birth of her son. The physicians were unable to control the bleeding and had to perform a hysterectomy (total removal of the uterus). I was frightened, but these doctors were only requiring a D&C. This news took Keith by surprise. He was confused and scared.

"Going under anesthesia so soon after having my baby was the worst part. I wasn't given an option for anesthesia. But I was also confused and took what they gave me. When I woke up, it took hours for me to recover. I felt very drowsy and rather insecure about handling the baby. I couldn't nurse Seth until 9:30 P.M. He was not nursing well. I was afraid he'd had too many bottles in the nursery.

"He went back to the nursery after that feeding because I still felt too drowsy to confidently handle him alone. By the 1:00 A.M. feeding, I was feeling better. The nurse brought him into my room and he stayed with me. My fears were allayed by this soft, comforting baby. Seth nursed and slept quietly. The following day we went home.

"Those first few days at home were difficult. I had left the hospital anemic with a hematocrit of 30% (normal is 42%). Just getting up in the morning and the activity of showering sent me back to bed for 1-2 hours. But I felt I could get more rest at home with my family than in the hospital. Keith was invaluable at this time. He helped with the laundry, cooking, and childcare. He even hired a housekeeper to clean the house for the first month.

"During these early days I rested as much as I could. I took lots of iron plus prenatal multiple vitamins as recommended by the nurse-midwife. Within a week's time, I had gained most of my strength back. After two weeks, I was almost back to normal. Six weeks after my hematocrit had returned to normal levels, and I once again embraced motherhood with renewed vigor."

AN EMERGENCY CESAREAN SECTION BIRTH

Mary is a PPF Master Teacher and a very good friend. She and her husband, Al, were in for quite a surprise during Kristin's birth.

Mary tells her story: "It was Monday morning and I had been having regular contractions since Saturday night. They weren't very strong and I'd only dilated three centimeters, so my midwife decided to break my bag of waters. This made my contractions much stronger. We all got really excited anticipating the birth. I drank two quarts of red raspberry leaf tea between Sunday night and Monday morning, trying to move my labor along. We must have walked around my block about twenty times. My baby, however, had other plans because my labor didn't progress much until about 8:00 Monday morning.

"That's when my contractions started to become really intense but not painful. Changing positions often is the key to having a pain-free labor. I was sure glad that I'd stayed flexible throughout my pregnancy by doing either the 'Salute to the Child' or the 'Basic Nine' every day. When I felt a contraction coming on, I'd get into a full squat and stay that way, breathing through the peak. Then I'd get into an all-fours position and rock or wiggle my seat, breathing until the contraction had ended. Until this labor,

I never believed that labor could be painless. Now I believe that every woman has to create her own 'Birth Dance' in order to gently aid her contractions in the process of getting the baby out.

"Soon I was going to move into the beautiful birth tub that my midwife and her brother-in-law had designed for maximum comfort during birthing. I had planned to spend late first and second stage labor there and to finally give birth to my baby peacefully in the warm water. We salted the water slightly to further simulate the intrauterine environment.

"After the midwife did an internal examination, those peaceful plans for a home birth had to be abandoned. Instead it was decided that we had to rush to the hospital. My baby had turned into a transverse position (sideways in the uterus) and wasn't moving. I was extremely disappointed that all our home birth plans would have to be changed. But I wanted more than anything to have a safe delivery and a healthy baby no matter what it took. At the hospital, the doctor confirmed that, because of the baby's position, an emergency Cesarean birth would be necessary.

"The doctor and the nursing staff could not have been more accommodating to us. I was first given an epidural that numbed me from the waist down, but I stayed wide awake! Both my husband and midwife came with me for support in the operating/ birthing room. The entire birth/operation took only about twenty minutes. I was in transition during the operation so my baby would have been born at the same time either way.

"The thing I remember most while being on the operating table was everyone commenting on the size of my baby. Kristin weighed nine pounds, three ounces. Right after I was sewn and stapled, and pictures were taken, everyone left Al, Kristin and me alone in one of the labor rooms for about half an hour. They even turned out the bright fluorescent lights to encourage our peacefulness in bonding.

"An hour after the birth, the IV of glucose water and pitocin that I had on was taken off. Then we all went up to my room. I was still holding my baby. Once we were settled, the midwife cleaned her up a bit at my bedside. After a while Al took her to the nursery to be weighed and to have her temperature taken. She was brought right back. When one of the nurses suggested an infant warmer for Kristin, I assured her that *I* was the best infant warmer my baby could have. Kristin saw the nursery only once more, while I had visitors in my room.

"Through gentle persuasion, the midwife got me out of bed and to the bathroom two hours after the birth. This was the best thing that she could have done for me. At the time, however, I thought that telling me to get out of bed and walking around was cruel and unusual treatment! I thought to myself, 'You want me to do *what* and walk *where*?' It was really difficult at first but I was glad that I was able to move around so quickly. When the post-operative gas pains came the next day, I was able to release them more easily than if I had stayed in bed. Other body movements I did those first two days included pointing and flexing my feet and deep, abdominal breathing ('Rock the Baby' breath).

"Al stayed with us all night for the two nights I was in the hospital. The nurses even brought him a cot to use. Not that either of us got much sleep. Since I couldn't do more than nurse Kristin and go to the bathroom, Al took care of changing diapers and walking with the baby. In addition, he helped me with many simple tasks that I couldn't yet perform.

"Kristin was born on Monday. On Wednesday, we were released from the hospital amid solemn promises to take our temperatures every few hours to make sure that neither of us developed infections. Much of my recovery was still ahead but I would definitely be more comfortable at home.

"My sister stayed with us until the end of the week to help Al with our other child, feeding, and housework. All I did was eat, sleep, and nurse for about a week. In other cultures, the newly-delivered mother is pampered as much as the new baby during the postpartum period. That is exactly how I felt! The most positive aspect of having a Cesarean birth is that I was forced to stay in a close family unit and just relax around the house. I don't think I would have reacted the same way had my second birth been a vaginal one. Al didn't go back to work for two and a half weeks after Kristin's birth.

"During this time, my state of mind changed frequently from sheer euphoria to sadness and self-doubt. About a week after the birth, I finally broke down and cried, mourning the death of my 'ideal birth.' A month later I'm still healing my body, mind and spirit from the shock of surgery. It really surprised me how much longer it took me to feel good again compared with my first daughter's vaginal birth.

"The third week after Kristin's birth, I was somewhat depressed. I was so sick of well-meaning people calling and opening the conversation with, 'I heard you had to have a C section.' I felt like screaming, 'I also had a beautiful baby girl!' That's what I thought they should have been more concerned with. I was still very tired and had to take a nap every day.

"At five weeks postpartum our family has adjusted fairly well to our new life. I owe my fast physical recovery to the fact that I remained in great condition throughout my pregnancy by teaching and practicing PPF and PPF WET. I feel good about my birth experience most of the time but I know that I still have some emotional healing to do. Talking to other women who have had Cesarean births helps.

"The most important thing I learned from this experience is to *stay forever flexible*. Although Kristin's birth was nothing like the birth I had planned, the experience was still enlightening, positive and exciting. Given the unpredictable nature of birth, you must remember that the most important person involved—the one who really determines what will ultimately happen—is the baby.

"Kristin is a big, beautiful, healthy and extremely peaceful baby. The ending to our little story could not have been happier."

A "VBAC" STORY (VAGINAL BIRTH AFTER CESAREAN)

Eileen and Patrick decided to try for a vaginal birth after Cesarean (or VBAC delivery) for the birth of their second child.

Eileen tells her story: "Our first child, Sarah, was born by Cesarean Section due to 'cephalopelvic disproportion' (CPD). My obstetricians explained that I had a small, protracted pelvis and that she was a large baby. In a way, I wasn't surprised because my mother had eight Cesarean births! Since we both have the same small build, I always assumed that I, too, would need surgery. It honestly didn't matter to me, though. My husband and I went through our Lamaze and PPF classes together, always hoping and praying for a healthy child no matter how he/she was born. I was in no way angry or bitter about having a Cesarean. I had a beautiful, healthy daughter!

"Three years later, I became pregnant with my second child. Throughout this pregnancy, people kept telling me that I didn't need another Cesarean just because I had one before. I knew that if I had surgery a second time, I would feel the same as after the first—tired but thrilled at the birth of my baby.

"In the meantime, two of my sisters had successful vaginal births, and I knew then that I wanted to try. Since surgery is obviously more dangerous than delivering vaginally, I felt I had an obligation to myself and my baby.

"My obstetricians felt I would be a good candidate for a VBAC. They explained that I would be prepared for surgery once labor had begun, 'just in case.' I appreciated that.

"The most difficult obstacle I had to overcome was fear. I kept asking myself if I was making the right choice. I knew what a Cesarean was like. Why not have another one? Could I really deliver vaginally, or would I need to have an emergency Cesarean at the last minute, after hours of painful labor?

"My obstetricians assured me that a non-progressive labor would not be allowed to continue for hours. If that were the case, the decision would be made to operate. I kept telling them that I wouldn't be disappointed if I needed another Cesarean!

"The one mistake I made during my second pregnancy was to attend a meeting of a support group for women who wanted to have a VBAC. I'm sure the kind of support given in this particular group is helpful to some women, but it certainly wasn't for me. The majority of women were extremely bitter about having a previous Cesarean. They were determined never to go through it again. I was virtually the only one in the group who felt I had had a positive birthing experience. Disappointment in having a Cesarean never entered my mind! The facilitator even hinted that I was headed for another Cesarean because I wasn't angry enough about the first!

"I left there feeling very sorry for those women, and extremely confused and depressed. Didn't they realize they were setting themselves up for disappointment and failure? I was determined not to get caught up in this way of thinking.

"My husband and I took a refresher course in Positive Pregnancy Fitness, which helped me tremendously, both physically and emotionally. The instructor confirmed what I already knew: I had a beautiful birthing experience the first time, and would again, no matter how the baby was born. A positive attitude is so very important! She helped me to re-learn breathing for control and relaxation. She recommended that I listen to some soothing music tapes during labor, which relaxed me a great deal.

"I began experiencing mild cramps at 9:00 A.M. and stayed home until 11:00 A.M., when contractions were five minutes apart. When I was admitted to the hospital at 11:30 A.M., the contractions were already three minutes apart, and I was 4 centimeters dilated. (I had only progressed to 2 centimeters with my first child.)

"For the next hour, I was told that my labor was progressing extremely well, although I was still frightened! At 12:35 P.M. I began pushing, and our son, James, was born at 12:45 P.M. weighing eight pounds, four ounces. The entire labor took less than four hours. We thanked God for a healthy little boy.

"Which birthing method did I prefer? Labor and delivery is not easy, no matter which birthing method is used. If I ever have a third child, we will again pray for a healthy one, no matter how he/she comes into the world!"

A FINAL NOTE

The birth of your baby can be a very exciting and joyous experience. The three weeks following the birth are often a time of adjustment and fatigue. You should find the following tips to be quite helpful:

- Try to have someone to help you (full time, if possible) during the first 1-2 weeks postpartum. This will enable you to rest and recuperate more quickly.
- Rest or sleep as much as you can at this time.
- Relieve engorged breasts by using a breast pump or by taking a hot shower.
- Keep taking your prenatal vitamins with iron.
- Eat 4-6 small nutritious meals a day.
- Snack and drink liquids often.
- Do PPF Abdominal Breathing to relax so that you can easily feed your baby.
- Have faith in yourself and your parenting abilities.

When you relive your child's birth, you will not always remember every detail. The experience often fades from memory. For this reason, I strongly recommend that you write down in detail all the events of this very important day in your life. In later years, it is fun to go back and mentally recall this very exciting day.

Appendix

PPF tapes, books and products are available to you through our mail-order company, *Be Healthy, Inc.* To order any of the products listed below, call or write:

> *Be Healthy, Inc.*
> 51 Saltrock Road
> Baltic, CT 06330
>
> 1-800-433-5523 (toll-free)
> In CT: 203-822-8573

We accept Mastercard and Visa. Please include $2.50 for shipping and handling. Allow 4-6 weeks for delivery. Also keep in mind that prices are subject to change. This is just a sampling of over 70 items that we stock.

If you have any personal inquiries, feel free to write to me, Sylvia Klein Olkin, at the above address. I'd be happy to hear from you.

PREGNANCY FITNESS TAPES

Positive Pregnancy Fitness
(by Sylvia Klein Olkin)

A quick, easy program for a trouble-free pregnancy.

- Innovative exercises and breathing techniques for eliminating lower backaches, side stitches and other complaints
- Washes away daily tensions, calms you down, reenergizes
- Narrated by Sylvia Klein Olkin with soothing background music
- Bond with your baby as it lives and strives within you
- Totally safe for any stage of pregnancy
- Includes an illustrated explanatory pamphlet

60 minute cassette/$11.95

Breathing for Birth
(by Sylvia Klein Olkin)

A unique, "breathe along" program.

- Best, most effective "breathing for birth" techniques (correlates with

the Lamaze Natural Childbirth program)
- Contains special controlled exhalation pushing techniques
- Contains exercises to strengthen the birth canal muscles for an easier birth and recuperation period
- Experience birth from the baby's viewpoint via unique relaxation/visualization
- Narrated by Sylvia Klein Olkin with soothing background music
- Includes an illustrated explanatory pamphlet

60 minute cassette/$11.95

Relax and Enjoy Your Baby Within
(by Sylvia Klein Olkin)

Bond with your baby as it's growing and flourishing inside you!

- Three separate 15-minute relaxation/visualizations especially designed for expectant Moms and Dads
- Relaxes, drains tension as you learn to tune into your inner child and your own inner strengths and abilities
- Narrated by Sylvia Klein Olkin with soothing background music
- Includes an instructional folder

45 minute cassette/$11.95

Any two of the above pregnancy tapes may be purchased for $22.00; all three pregnancy tapes may be purchased for $31.00.

PREGNANCY AND BIRTH BOOKS

Transformation Through Birth: A Woman's Guide (Bergin and Garvey, 1984) by Claudia Panuthos

An exhilarating combination of knowledgeable research and the collective wisdom of thousands of women and birthing couples. Also contains information on the use of visualization during pregnancy and birth.

191 pages/$12.95

The Secret Life of the Unborn Child: Prepare Your Unborn Baby for a Happy, Healthy Life (A Delta Book, 1981) by Thomas Verny, M.D., with John Kelly

Life before birth—will your child remember? This book tells you what your unborn is capable of before birth. Change your experience of pregnancy and childbirth forever! (See *Love Chords* under "Other Pregnancy Products.")

253 pages/$8.95

Silent Knife: Cesarean Prevention and Vaginal Birth After Cesarean (Bergin and Garvey, 1983) by Nancy Wainer Cohen and Lois Estner

A thoroughly researched book written in a lively, humorous manner on the escalating Cesarean rate in this country and how to avoid the operation initially, or how to have a vaginal birth after a Cesarean. Contains touching personal accounts from women all over the United States.

435 pages/$14.95

The Brewer Medical Diet for Normal and High-Risk Pregnancy (Simon and Schuster, 1983) by Gail Sforza Brewer

The first authoritative book to provide the expectant mother with a specific, proper nutritional-management program. Covers problems ranging from cramps to toxemia. Written in an easy-to-understand, "question and answer" manner. Also contains vegetarian diets for pregnancy.

244 pages/$8.95

To Baby With Love: Your Prenatal Food Diary (Bull Publishing, 1982) by Marilyn Hanson, M.S., and Robert Sefura, R.N.

Clear, accurate information on optimum pregnancy nutrition; delicious recipes; a daily food diary; plus space to record your thoughts and feelings throughout the pregnancy, and to share with your child in the future!

300 pages/$9.95

Pregnant Fathers (Prentice-Hall, 1982) by Jack Heinowitz

A text for fathers that describes how they can enjoy and share the experience of pregnancy and birth. The perfect gift for the expectant father.

126 pages/$6.95

OTHER PREGNANCY PRODUCTS

Positive Pregnancy Fitness Maternity T-Shirt

Great for lounging and exercise! White 50/50 Cotton/Poly blends scoop neck, cap sleeve with *Positive Pregnancy Fitness* logo on upper left in kelly green with hot pink hearts. Something every woman should own!

S, M, L, and XL/$17.00

Almond Glow Skin Lotion

Calming massage oil. An Edgar Cayce formulation. Use as a massage oil, suntan oil, or bath oil. Can be used for prenatal nipple preparation prior to breastfeeding. Helps to relieve discomfort of stretchmarks. Contains all natural ingredients:

pure peanut oil, virgin olive oil, lanolin oil, almond oil, and vitamin E. Comes in either a light flourishing almond or coconut musk scent.

2 oz./$2.50 (almond scent only)
8 oz./$6.50

Red Raspberry Leaf/Organic Herbal Tea

The most recommended tea for pregnancy, childbirth and postpartum. Helps to eliminate nausea, prepares the uterus for labor and birth. The best-known herbal aid! Also includes "The Red Raspberry Leaf Story."

1 oz./$1.25
2 oz./$2.25

Love Chords
(by Thomas R. Verny, M.D.)

Music to promote "inner bonding." Stimulates and enhances the emotional and intellectual development of your unborn child. Contains classical music selections that babies in utero seem to enjoy. A fun way to bond with your baby when it is still in the womb. Also includes an instruction folder that charts your baby's development from a week to nine months prior to the birth, and tips on how to use *Love Chords* for a super pregnancy.

40 minute cassette/$10.00

Seiza Bench

Here's help for the pregnant woman. The seiza bench enables her to sit up straight without any strain. Excellent for women with varicose veins. Handcrafted from premium grades of native hardwood. These compact benches measure 7" × 17" on top and 8" high in back. Includes an introductory pamphlet.

$20.00 (add an extra $2.50 for shipping and handling)

PARENTING PRODUCTS

Shape Up With Baby
(by Sylvia Klein Olkin)

Regain your pre-pregnancy shape (or an even better one!)

- •Exercise and shape up with your new baby
- •Flatten your tummy and slim your hips, thighs, buttocks, and waist
- •Eliminate tensions and revitalize your mind and body
- •Special exercises just for baby
- •Includes an illustrated pamphlet

60 minute cassette/$11.95

Practical Parenting Tips (Simon and Schuster, 1980) by Vicki Lansky

For parents who want to save time, trouble, money and make life easier. Contains over 1000 ideas for new parents for the first five years. A life-saving book that all parents should have on hand at all times.

164 pages/$6.95

Infant Massage: A Handbook for Loving Parents (A Bantam Book, 1982) by Vimala Schneider

Discusses sharing and communicating love to your newborn through massage. This book helps to enhance the bond between you and your infant and gives the father the contact he often misses. Easy, enjoyable reading.

125 pages/$5.95

NEW BABY PRODUCTS

Happy Family Breast Pump

The cadillac of hand breast pumps. A pain-free, totally effective pump that will help breastfeeding mothers to collect milk for later feedings, relieve engorged breasts, and enable working mothers to breastfeed. It is constructed of non-breakable plastic and can be sterilized in the dishwasher.

- •American-made pump features two sizes for breast cups
- •Angles down from the body for comfort and easy use so that milk doesn't spill
- •Unit converts into a bottle with an orthodontic nipple

$22.00 (add $2.50 for shipping and handling)

Free and Dry Breast Care Shields

Eliminates stains from milk leakage, helps correct inverted nipples, helps relieve cracked nipples. Feather-light flesh plastic tint shield worn over breasts inside bra to collect and contain milk leakage. Comes with its own carrying case.

$7.00 per pair

MUSIC TO INDUCE RELAXATION

Sweet Baby Dreams
(by Steven Bergman)

Music to calm babies, children and expectant mothers. Lullaby music is incorporated with a pregnant mother's heartbeat. Great for relaxing and quieting the newborn.

40 minute cassette/$10.00

Slumberland
(by Steven Bergman)

Natural, uplifting tempo that gradually

moves to a soothing melody. Music by flute, guitar, string orchestra, and synthesizer are combined with sounds of birds, crickets, and heartbeats. A must for all parents who wish to calm their baby's environment.

40 minute cassette/$10.00

Lullabies From Around The World
(by Steve Bergman)

An orchestral interpretation of gentle lullabies from around the world. Calming for mothers, babies and children of all ages. Also helpful in reducing stress and quieting one's surroundings. A favorite of ours and soon to be yours.

Specially Priced: $10.00

Comfort Zone
(by Steven Halpren)

Bathes the listener in a warm caress of sound. The feeling is that of a lullaby orchestrated on keyboards and softly sustaining strings.

40 minute cassette/$10.00

Spectrum Suite
(by Steven Halpren)

Triggers a state of relaxation and enhances awareness. Side One features the warm sounds of electronic piano; Side Two adds exquisite ensemble settings.

40 minute cassette/$10.00

Eventide
(by Steven Halpern)

Piano music on Side One; soothing electronic music featuring lullaby melodies on Side Two. Great for the newborn.

40 minute cassette/$10.00

You Are The Ocean
(by Schawkie Roth)

Perfect music for relaxation, meditation, or simply feeling joyful! Celestial water music is created by blending the sounds of the ocean or stream with flute, harp, cello, and zither in the background. Harmonious melodies interweave with oriental flowing bamboo and alto flutes.

40 minute cassette/$10.00

Piano Means Soft
(by Charley Thweatt)

This tape promotes a gentle, flowing, peaceful inner calm. Moves you to a quiet state of being. The gentle acoustics and electronic piano help to induce relaxation.

40 minute cassette/$10.00

Glossary

Anal muscles. The muscles that open and close the rectal outlet.

Anemia. A condition in which the red corpuscles of the blood are reduced in number or are deficient in hemoglobin.

Anus. The muscular outlet of the rectum (lower end of the large intestine).

Asanas. Yoga postures, poses, or movements. Literally translated from Sanskrit, it means easy, firm, steady position.

Baby Breath. A special breathing technique that facilitates inner bonding and helps to prepare for the pushing stage of labor.

Birth canal. The vagina, through which the baby passes at birth.

Birth mandala. A geometric design that has been especially created for you to use as an outward focus during labor and delivery. *See also* Mandala.

Bloody show. The mucous plug (often tinged with blood) that is released from the cervix before or during early labor.

Braxton-Hicks contractions. Physical contractions of the uterus that occur throughout pregnancy, which prepare the uterus for labor.

Cervix. The lowest, bottleneck-shaped portion of the uterus that opens into the vagina or birth canal.

Cesarean birth. The birth of a baby using surgical incisions either in the abdominal or pubic area.

Chakra (chuk'ruh). A Sanskrit word meaning "internal energy center of the body." There are seven energy centers, according to yogic theory.

Colostrum. The first fluid secreted by the mother's breasts before her milk arrives. It is high in antibodies and protein.

Contraction. A tensing or shortening of the muscle fibers of the uterus, which is followed by a relaxation or lengthening of these fibers.

Crowning. The visual appearance of the baby's head at the vaginal or birth canal outlet.

Diaphragm. A large, thick muscle that separates the chest (thorax) from the abdomen. This is the muscle used in "Rock the Baby" breath.

Dilatation. The opening of the cervix during the first stage of labor. Is always measured in centimeters.

Edema. Bodily swelling caused by excess fluid retained by the body's tissues.

Effacement. The thinning of the cervix prior to or during labor.

Episiotomy. A surgical incision or cut, usually made with scissors, of the perineum (outer birth canal) to give the baby's head more room, prevent tearing of the vagina, and make the birth smoother.

Fetus. A medical term for the baby as it grows inside from the third month to the end of the pregnancy.

Hemorrhoids. Inflamed and often painful veins of the rectum.

In utero. "Within the uterus."

Intravenous infusion (IV). Fluids or medication administered through the vein via a needle and drip bottle.

Lactation. The secretion or formation of milk, or the period of milk production in the female body.

Lightening. The descent of the baby into the pelvis.

Lochia. Vaginal discharge after delivery.

Mandala (mun dah'luh). The Sanskrit word for "circle" or "center." It consists of a series of concentric forms. In many cultures the mandala symbolizes the entire cosmos, and the dot placed within it represents the essence or the source of things. It is used for centering and concentration.

Mantras (muhn'truz). The sacred words and sounds that have been used in Eastern countries for centuries for healing and spiritual development.

Meditation. The relaxation of the body and the quieting of the mind during concentration on the breath, or an internal or external sound.

Midwife. A person who assists women in childbirth.

Miscarriage. The loss of the baby before the end of the seventh month of pregnancy.

Om (ohm). The highest mantra; the vibration of life energy.

Pelvic floor. Muscle layers that form a sling across the base of the pelvis and support the bladder, uterus, and rectum.

Pelvis. The bones that form the two hip bones, the sacrum, and the tailbone.

Perineum. The area between the anus and the external genitals.

Placenta. An organ that nourishes the unborn child via the umbilical cord throughout the pregnancy. After the baby is born, the placenta is also expelled and called the afterbirth.

Postpartum. The period of time, following the birth of the baby, before the mother returns to her pre-pregnancy condition.

Prenatal. The time period during pregnancy before the baby is born.

Quickening. The first movements of the fetus felt by the mother. Usually occurs between the sixteenth and twentieth weeks of growth.

"Rock the Baby" Breath. Yogic abdominal breathing to be used throughout all the pregnancy months.

Root chakra. The first basic energy center of the body located between the anus and the genital area.

Round ligaments. Fibrous muscles connecting the uterus and the pelvic bones.

Supine position. Any posture that begins while lying flat on the back.

Umbilical cord. The physical connection that supplies the unborn baby with its nourishment. It contains two arteries and one vein to exchange oxygen, nutrients, and waste products between the placenta and the baby.

Urethra. The narrow passageway through which urine is discharged from the bladder.

Uterus. The womb in which the baby grows during the nine months of pregnancy.

Vagina. The muscular birth canal leading from the uterus to the outer genitals.

Varicose veins. Swollen, painful veins, usually of the legs, but often in the genitals, too.

Yin and Yang. In Chinese thought, the complementary forces that pervade the universe. The interaction of these two forces causes things to happen.

Yoga (yo'guh). A Sanskrit word meaning "to yoke or fasten together." A scientific system for bringing about a natural balance in the mind, body, and spirit.

Bibliography

BREASTFEEDING

La Leche League International. *The Womanly Art of Breastfeeding*, revised edition, 1981.

A very thorough guide to breastfeeding by the organization that has been counseling nursing mothers for over 25 years. Good factual information. Supports and encourages full-time mothering.

Presser, Janet, Brewer, Gail, and Freehand, Julianna. *Breastfeeding*, 1983.

A beautifully illustrated book that provides guidance on everything from how to begin nursing to ways of weaning.

Pryor, Karen. *Nursing Your Baby*, 1973.

A well-written guide for new nursing mothers.

CESAREAN BIRTH

C/Sec, Inc. *Frankly Speaking: A Pamphlet for Cesarean Couples*. Call or write: 22 Forest Rd., Framingham, MA 01701; (617) 542-2004. Cost is $4.25.

A pamphlet that explains the reasons for a C/Sec.

Cohen, Nancy Wainer, and Estner, Lois J. *Silent Knife: Cesarean Prevention and Vaginal Delivery After Cesarean*, 1983.

A thoroughly researched and easy-to-read book on the escalating Cesarean section rate in this country and how to avoid the operation initially, or how to have a vaginal birth after a Cesarean. Contains personal accounts from women all over the country. Written in a lively, factual, and often humorous manner that can help every pregnant couple to learn about their options. Highly recommended. (Available through PPF; see the Appendix.)

Duffy, Cynthia, and Meyer, Linda. *Responsible Childbirth: How to Give Birth Normally—And Avoid a Cesarean Section*, 1984.

235

Details choosing a birth attendant and facility, Cesarean prevention techniques, vaginal birth after Cesarean, and much more. Recommended.

Norwood, Christopher. *How to Avoid a Cesarean Section*, 1984.

Explains strategies used to avert unnecessary surgery and procedures available to obtain the best medical care if surgery is needed.

Wilson, Christine Coleman, and Hovey, Wendy Roe. *Cesarean Childbirth: A Handbook for Parents*, 1981.

An invaluable resource for couples to prepare themselves for all the possibilities of childbirth. Contents range from trends and issues in obstetrics to parent-infant bonding.

CHILDBIRTH

Ashford, Janet Isaacs. *Birth Stories: The Experience Remembered*, 1984.

Childbirth is remembered at home and in the hospital in 34 different birth stories. Should be of particular interest to women who are pregnant for the first time and those who have felt isolated by a difficult birth.

Bing, Elizabeth. *Six Practical Lessons for an Easier Childbirth*, revised edition, 1982.

A step-by-step Lamaze guide by a well-known childbirth educator. Standard reading when taking Lamaze classes.

Brewer, Gail, and Greene, Janice Presser. *Right From The Start*, 1981.

Provides information and support for women who want to experience child-

birth in the most natural way possible. Recommended.

Dick-Read, Grantly. *Childbirth Without Fear*, 1972.

A wonderful book by the originator of prepared childbirth. Contains a good discussion of the relationship between relaxation and an easier labor and birth. Recommended.

Feldman, Sylvia. *Choices in Childbirth*, 1978.

A thorough, well-organized, and practical approach to the alternatives in childbirth. Includes sections on hospital birth and home birth with a midwife. A good book with basic information.

Fenlon, Arlene, McPherson, Ellen, and Dorchak, Lovell. *Getting Ready for Childbirth*, revised edition, 1986.

An excellent guidebook on all aspects of pregnancy and birth. Some information on postpartum is provided as well. Highly recommended.

Kitzinger, Sheila. *The Complete Book of Pregnancy and Childbirth*, 1980.

A comprehensive guide to pregnancy and childbirth. Fully illustrated with photographs, drawings, and diagrams. Highly recommended.

Kitzinger, Sheila. *Experience of Childbirth*, third edition, 1984.

A top-notch book on the many aspects of pregnancy and birth written by a famous British childbirth educator. Takes the human aspect into account. Highly recommended.

Leboyer, Frederick. *Birth Without Violence*, 1975.

A book about a quiet, peaceful, respectful birth for your baby using the Leboyer method. Beautifully written and illustrated with sensitive photos. Highly recommended.

Lesko, Wendy and Matthew. *The Maternity Sourcebook*, 1984.

An exhaustive exploration of factors in childbirth and early child care to help parents to make their own decisions concerning pregnancy, delivery, and baby care. Highly recommended.

Panuthos, Claudia. *Transformation Through Birth: A Woman's Guide*, 1984.

Knowledgeable research and collective wisdom from the experiences of thousands of women and birthing couples. Chapters on preparation for birth using visualizations and release. Highly recommended. (Available through PPF; see the Appendix.)

Peterson, Gayle H. *Birthing Normally: A Personal Growth Approach to Childbirth*, second edition, 1984.

Insight on approaching prenatal care. Incorporates holistic concepts to maximize women's chances of giving birth normally without intervention.

Samuels, Michael, M.D., and Nancy. *The Well Pregnancy Book*, 1986.

Gives a holistic understanding of pregnancy and birth so that parents can make satisfactory choices. Recommended.

Simkin, Penny, Whalley, Janet, and Keppler, Ann. *Pregnancy, Childbirth and the Newborn: A Complete Guide for Expectant Parents*, 1983.

An indispensable guide for expectant and new parents. Covers nutrition, prenatal procedures, health care providers, birth places, exercise, and relaxation with a strong presentation of parental choices. Highly recommended.

COOKBOOKS

Katzen, Mollie. *The Enchanted Broccoli Forest*, 1982.

More creative recipes from Mrs. Katzen. This book includes a chapter devoted to bread baking. Highly recommended.

Katzen, Mollie. *Moosewood Cookbook*, 1977.

A beautifully illustrated, creative vegetarian cookbook based on the recipes used at the Moosewood Restaurant in Ithaca, NY. The variety, ingenuity, and tastiness of the recipes make this book a must to own if you want to learn more about vegetarian cooking. Highly recommended.

Lappe, Frances Moore. *Diet for a Small Planet*, revised edition, 1984.

The sourcebook on complementary proteins. An excellent discussion of how incomplete proteins can be combined to produce high-grade protein nutrition. Also contains a variety of recipes to put these ideas into practice.

Robertson, Laurel, Flinders, Carol, and Godfrey, Bronwen. *Laurel's Kitchen*, revised edition, 1987.

A complete reference book for vegetarian cooking. Contains a huge variety of recipes and is written in a folksy manner.

Also includes thorough nutritional charts. Highly recommended.

EXERCISE

Balaskas, Arthur and Janet. *New Life: The Book of Exercises for Childbirth*, revised edition, 1983.

This beautiful, creative, and highly educational book presents the British viewpoint of prepared childbirth. Highly recommended.

Dale, Barbara, and Roeber, Johanna. *The Pregnancy Exercise Book*, 1982.

A joyful book about body awareness in pregnancy, nicely illustrated with luscious photos.

Noble, Elisabeth. *Essential Exercises for the Childbearing Year*, revised edition, 1982.

Well-explained exercises and extensive text on pregnancy and postpartum. Includes rehabilitation after a C-section. Nicely illustrated with line drawings. Recommended.

FOR FATHERS

Dodson, Fitzhugh. *How to Father*, 1975.

Concerns children from birth to twenty-one years of age. Recommended for mothers as well as fathers.

Heinowitz, Jack. *Pregnant Fathers*, 1982.

Examines the feelings, needs, and concerns of expectant and new fathers. Highly recommended. (Available through PPF; see the Appendix.)

Sullivan, S. Adams. *The Father's Almanac*, 1980.

A practical book about fatherhood with ideas on how to spend "quality time" with your child, from babyhood to preschool.

HEALTH

Berkeley Holistic Health Center. *The Holistic Health Handbook*, 1978.

A sourcebook of the many approaches to health. Includes articles on Oriental systems, Native American systems, Western systems, as well as the techniques and practices of holistic health. A good reference book on the newest approaches to total health.

Boston Women's Health Book Collective. *The New Our Bodies, Our Selves*, revised edition, 1985.

Totally revised with new information on pregnancy. Written by women to help other women to understand themselves better. A really good sourcebook.

Bricklin, Mark. *The Practical Encyclopedia of Natural Healing*, 1983.

This encyclopedia covers virtually every common illness and every important natural healing modality that offers genuine benefits. Also contains an index for pregnancy.

Kepit, Wynn, and Elson, Lawrence M. *The Anatomy Coloring Book*, 1977.

Learn about the inner workings of your body by coloring each section. A good way to have fun as you learn.

Samuels, Michael, M.D., and Bennett, Hal. *The Well Body Book*, revised edition, 1984.

How to use the healing energy that your body possesses. A very good sourcebook for learning more about how your body works or breaks down. Recommended.

HERBS

Hylton, William H., ed. *The Rodale Herb Book; How to Use, Grow, and Buy Nature's Miracle Plants*, 1978.

A sourcebook on herbs and their uses.

Koehler, Nan Ullrike. *Artemis Speaks: With VBAC Stories and Natural Childbirth Information*, 1985.

A sourcebook of information on herbs and their uses during pregnancy and postpartum. With over 500 pages, this book was written by a botanist and herbologist. It is printed in large type, and is easy to read and understand. Very highly recommended.

Thomson, Robert. *Natural Medicine*, 1978.

Contains specific herbal recommendations for labor and delivery, as well as an account of the author's wife's use of herbs at the time of their child's birth.

Weed, Susan S. *Wise Woman Herbal for the Childbearing Year*, 1985.

Contains specific herbal recommendations for pregnancy and postpartum. It is very well organized and contains chapters on Herbs Before Pregnancy, Herbs During Pregnancy, Herbs After Pregnancy, Your Infant, and the Herbal Pharmacy. Recommended.

HOME BIRTH

Baldwin, Rahima. *Special Delivery: The*

Complete Guide to Informed Birth, revised edition, 1986.

A practical guide for couples who want to take greater responsibility for the births of their babies. Recommended.

Gaskin, Ina May. *Spiritual Midwifery*, revised edition, 1980.

Inspiring accounts of birth at *The Farm*, a self-sufficient farming community in Tennessee. Provides advice on both the spiritual and physical aspects of childbirth preparation and parenting.

Sousa, Marion. *Childbirth at Home*, 1977.

A complete discussion of the pros and cons of home birth. Must reading for any couple considering home birth.

White, Gregory J., M.D. *Emergency Childbirth*, 1976.

A factual handbook for emergency birth situations. Well worth reading.

MASSAGE

Downing, George. *The Massage Book*, revised edition, 1981.

A good basic book on massage strokes and techniques. Well illustrated.

Inkeles, Gordon. *Massage and Peaceful Pregnancy*, 1983.

An essential guide for all expectant parents concerning the benefits of massage during childbearing.

Leboyer, Frederick. *Loving Hands: The Traditional Indian Art of Baby Massage*, 1976.

Beautiful prose, photographs, and feelings pervade this instructive book on baby massage.

Ohasi, Waturu and Hoover, Mary. *Shiatsu For A Healthy Pregnancy and Delivery*, 1984.

A thoroughly-explained guide to Shiatsu, or pressure point therapy, during pregnancy and labor. Leads the reader step by step through a Shiatsu session. Recommended.

Schneider, Vimala. *Infant Massage*, 1982.

A clearly-illustrated guide to massaging your baby, including songs to sing and games to play. Highly recommended. (Available through PPF; see the Appendix.)

MEDITATION

Peck, Robert L. *American Meditation and Beginning Yoga*, 1976.

A clear, well-written, scientific approach and explanation of Raja Yoga, as well as altered states of consciousness. (Available through PPF; send for our catalog.)

Peck, Robert L. and Thelma. *The Path: Between Cosmos and Created*, 1985.

An essential part of the teaching of yoga is the goal for which each individual strives. *The Path* provides a guide one can follow to achieve that goal. (Available through PPF; send for our catalog.)

Dass, Ram. *The Journey of Awakening: A Meditator's Guidebook*, 1978.

Contains information on meditation as well as a state-by-state listing of available meditation groups. It is a good source for those students wishing to find other meditators. Highly recommended.

NUTRITION

Brewer, Gail Sforza. *The Brewer Medical Diet for Normal and High Risk Pregnancy*, 1983.

Provides a specific, proper nutritional counseling program for every stage of pregnancy and after. Written in an easy-to-understand manner. Highly recommended. (Available through PPF; see the Appendix.)

Brewer, Tom and Gail. *What Every Pregnant Woman Should Know: The Truth About Diets and Drugs in Pregnancy*, revised edition, 1986.

Carefully explains the relationship between good nutrition and having a healthy baby and a positive pregnancy. Also has a good discussion of toxemia. (Available through PPF; send for our catalog).

California Department of Health Services. *Nutrition During Pregnancy and Lactation*, 714-744 P Street, Sacramento, CA 95814.

A research report on the nutritional requirements of different ethnic groups. Has good daily intake guidelines.

Elliot, Rose. *The Vegetarian Mother and Baby Book*, 1986.

Gives nutrition information and recipes for pregnancy, breastfeeding and post-weaning.

Goldbeck, Nikki. *As You Eat So Your Baby Grows*, revised edition, 1986.

This well-illustrated pamphlet is must reading for all pregnant women. Concisely explains what should be part of a balanced prenatal diet. Available for $2.50 from : CERES PRESS, Box 87, Woodstock, NY 12498. Highly recommended.

Lansky, Vicki. *The Taming of the C.A.N.D.Y. Monster (Continuously Advertised, Nutritionally Deficient Yummies)*, 1977.

A guide for eliminating or minimizing your child's consumption of junk food. Has good ideas for high nutrition snacks, desserts, etc. Good for pre-school and elementary school children.

National Academy of Sciences National Research Council, Food and Nutrition Board. *Recommended Dietary Allowances*, revised edition, 1985.

The latest findings of minimum daily requirements of nutrients, vitamins, and minerals.

Nutrition Search, Inc. *Nutrition Almanac*, revised edition, 1984.

A basic book on understanding nutrition. Has comprehensive charts on the vitamin, mineral, and caloric content of numerous foods. Recommended.

U.S. Department of Agriculture. *Handbook of the Nutritional Contents of Foods*, revised edition, 1982.

Contains complete charts of the nutritive values of an extensive variety of foods. A good book for discovering what's in the food you eat.

U.S. Department of Health, Education, and Welfare. *Alcohol and Your Unborn Child*, revised edition, 1985.

Must reading for every pregnant woman. Discusses the latest findings on how alcohol affects the unborn child.

Williams, Phyllis, R.N. *Nourishing Your Unborn Child*, revised edition, 1982.

A basic book on nutrition that can help during pregnancy. Has a variety of appetizing recipes.

ORGANIZATIONS

American College of Nurse-Midwives (ACNM)
1522 K. St. NW. #110
Washington, DC 20005

ACNM establishes and maintains standards for the practice of nurse-midwifery and can refer you to certified nurse-midwives practicing in your area.

American College of Obstetricians and Gynecologists (ACOG)
Resource Center
600 Maryland Ave., SW
Washington, DC 20024

ACOG sets national standards in obstetrical education and practice; free copies of a number of patient-information booklets are available on such topics as alcohol during pregnancy.

American Foundation for Maternal and Child Health
30 Beekman Pl.
New York, NY 10022

This foundation, headed by Doris Haire, acts as a clearinghouse on birth practices and makes pamphlets available. Write to inquire about the literature that is offered.

ASPO/Lamaze
1840 Wilson Blvd. #204
Arlington, VA 22201

The American Society of Psycho-prophylaxis in Obstetrics promotes the Lamaze method of prepared childbirth and sponsors a nationally-standardized teacher certification program.

Birth and Life Bookstore
PO Box 7-625
Seattle, WA 98107

A mail-order house specializing in books on pregnancy and postpartum. It carries hundreds of titles, many of which can no longer be purchased at your local bookstore. Write for a free copy of their super catalog.

Cesarean Prevention Movement (CPM)
PO Box 152
Syracuse, NY 13210

CPM is dedicated to lowering the Cesarean section rate, which has an alarming 20% rate in the U.S. It also encourages vaginal birth after a Cesarean. CPM sponsors classes on how to avoid a Cesarean, and you can write to them for further information.

Cesarean/Support, Education, Concern (C/ SEC)
22 Forest Road
Farmington, MA 01701

C/SEC publishes booklets on a range of topics, including father-attended Cesarean birth.

Informed Birth and Parenting Bookstore
501 Berkeley Ave.
Ann Arbor, MI 48103

This mail-order bookstore specializes in

publications and manuals for those planning a home birth.

International Childbirth Education Association (ICEA)
PO Box 20048
Minneapolis, MN 55420

ICEA is an interdisciplinary organization that operates a mail-order bookstore and publishes a newsletter and numerous pamphlets on maternal and newborn care. Write to them and add your name to their mailing list.

La Leche League International (LLLI)
9616 Minneapolis Ave.
Franklin Park, IL 60131

LLLI has local chapters throughout the United States and breastfeeding support groups for mothers. A newsletter and other literature is available for non-members.

Mothers of Twins
5402 Amberwood Lane
Rockville, MD 20803

This organization is devoted to making things easier for mothers of twins. Write to them for a publication list.

National Association of Parents and Professionals for Safe Alternatives in Childbirth (NAPSAC)
PO Box 646
Marble Hill, MO 63764

NAPSAC publishes such books as *Twenty-First Century Obstetrics Now!* and is concerned about obstetrical interventions and hospital practice.

National Foundation of the March of Dimes
Public Health Education Dept.

1275 Mamaroneck Ave.
White Plains, NY 10605

The March of Dimes distributes free pamphlets and fact sheets on such concerns as birth defects, prematurity, and toxoplasmosis. A catalog is available.

Nurse's Association of the American College of Obstetricians and Gynecologists (NAACOG)
600 Maryland Ave. SW
Washington, DC 20024

NAACOG may be able to help you find local childbirth preparation groups and other resources.

Orange Cat
442 Church St.
Garberville, CA 95440

This mail-order bookstore carries titles on birth and parenting.

Positive Pregnancy and Parenting Fitness
51 Saltrock Road
Baltic, CT 06330

Trains and certifies PPF teachers throughout the United States. Has books, tapes, videotapes, and other childbirth-related information. Send a business-sized, self-addressed, stamped envelope for a copy of the latest catalog and teacher training workshop schedule.

The Pre- and Peri-Natal Psychology Association of North America (PPPANA)
c/o Dr. Thomas Verny
36 Madison Ave.
Toronto, Ontario
Canada M5R 2S1

PPPANA is dedicated to exploring and developing an understanding of the unborn and newborn child. Prenatal Psychology is a brand new field that can contribute much understanding to the factors influencing mothers and fathers during pregnancy. For membership application, which entitles you to a quarterly newsletter and other research data, write to Dr. Verny.

PARENTING

Fraiberg, Selma. *The Magic Years*, 1959.

Provides excellent insight into the interior life of the infant and young child. Highly recommended.

Javitch, Karen, and Freidman, Amy. *Mother Knows Best*, 1982.

Hints contributed by mothers across the United States on many aspects of the first four years of life. Covers bathing, feeding, safety, travel, first-aid, and much more.

Rakowitz, Elly, and Rubin, Gloria. *Living With Your New Baby: A Postpartum Guide For Mothers and Fathers*, 1978.

A good description of feelings and situations in early parenthood.

Spock, Benjamin, and Rothenberg, Michael. *Dr. Spock's Baby and Child Care*, revised edition, 1985.

The handbook for knowing when to call the doctor if your child is sick. Useful for detecting the symptoms of an illness and gaining a better understanding of your growing child. Recommended.

PARENTING MAGAZINES

American Baby, 325 Evelyn St., Paramus, NJ 07652.

Features articles on prenatal and infant care, nursery planning ideas, maternity fashions, and more. Send a postcard to the above address for a free subscription.

Baby Talk, 185 Madison Ave., New York, NY 10016. Subscription: $6.75/year.

This monthly magazine contains brief, general interest articles for new parents.

Mothering, PO Box 8410, Santa Fe, NM 87504. Subscription: $15.00/year.

A wonderful and touching magazine with articles written by mothers relating their feelings, experiences, etc. Well worth reading and saving.

POSTPARTUM

Lansky, Vicki. *Practical Parenting Tips*, 1982.

Contains trouble, time, and money-saving ideas. Highly recommended. (Available through PPF; see the Appendix.)

Rozdilsky, Marylou, and Banet, Barbara. *What Now? A Handbook of New Parents Postpartum*, revised edition, 1975.

A straightforward, often funny, guidebook for new parents. Contains information on physical changes after birth, sex, depression, shared responsibilities, etc. Highly recommended.

PREGNANCY

Bing, Elizabeth, and Colman, Libby. *Making Love During Pregnancy*, 1977.

A clear, straightforward, and honest discussion of the interrelationship between pregnancy and sexuality. Well illustrated with beautiful line drawings.

Should be required reading for all parents-to-be. Highly recommended.

Brewer, Gail Sforza. *The Pregnancy After Thirty Workbook*, 1978.

A positive approach to childbearing in the thirties. Includes a variety of articles on diet, self-awareness, and exercise for a trouble-free birth and postpartum period. Also contains a limited exercise section.

Hotchner, Tracy. *Pregnancy and Childbirth*, revised edition, 1984.

An encyclopedia on pregnancy, breast-feeding, and postpartum. Contains good factual information, but is lacking in organization.

Montagu, Ashley. *Life Before Birth*, 1977.

An exciting exploration of the world of the prenatal child and how the mother affects and interacts with it. Recommended.

PRENATAL PSYCHOLOGY

Verny, Thomas, M.D. *The Secret Life of the Unborn Child*, 1981.

Deals with the phenomena of the unborn and how language, music, and other environmental factors affect the fetus in utero. Also discusses the direct impact that Mom's emotions have on the child. Highly recommended. (Available through PPF; see the Appendix.)

PSYCHOLOGICAL ASPECTS OF PREGNANCY

Jimenez, Sherry. *Childbearing: A Guide For Pregnant Parents*, 1980.

Contains a practical and thorough

chapter on the emotional aspects of pregnancy.

Kitzinger, Sheila. *The Experience of Childbirth*, third edition, 1984.

Particular focus is on the psychological aspects of pregnancy. Highly recommended.

Stern, Sue Ellen. *Expecting Change: The Emotional Journey Through Pregnancy*, 1986.

Enables the mother-to-be to experience greater fulfillment through understanding her emotions.

RELAXATION

Benson, Herbert. *The Relaxation Response*, revised edition, 1982.

A clear, scientific understanding of how to learn how to relax.

White, John, and Fadiman, James. *Relax: How You Can Feel Better, Reduce Stress, and Overcome Tension*, 1976.

Explores a variety of approaches for inducing relaxation. A good book for better understanding the relaxation response.

YOGA

Folan, Lilias M. *Lilias, Yoga and Your Life*, 1981.

A well-illustrated guide to beginning Hatha Yoga by television yoga teacher, Lilias.

Staff of the Kripalu Center. *The Self-Health Guide*, 1983.

An excellent introduction to yoga and how you can use different techniques to achieve a radiant state of well-being. To get on their mailing list, write: Kripalu Shop, Box 774, Dept. M., Lenox, MA 01240.

Zebroff, Kareen. *The ABC of Yoga*, 1979.

An organized and informative book for beginning yoga students. Contains numerous photos and is highly recommended.

About the Author

Sylvia Klein Olkin has a Masters degree in Education/Eastern Studies and is currently the director of *Positive Pregnancy and Parenting Fitness*. She has been teaching prenatal fitness classes since 1975 and has been training other qualified women to teach the PPF program since 1980. She has appeared on numerous talk shows on radio and television, and recently returned from China, where she introduced the *Positive Pregnancy Fitness* program to Chinese childbirth educators.

Index to Exercises

General Index